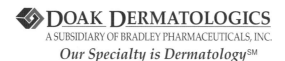

Doak Dermatologics is proud to sponsor this original photographic dermatology educational series, *Photographic History of Nineteenth Century Dermatology*. Please enjoy Volume 2, *The Torso*, with our compliments.

From the first publications on the treatment of skin diseases in the 1830s, medical research in the specialty of dermatology has produced innovative treatments for numerous skin diseases, improving health and quality of life for millions of patients.

The Burns Archive includes a remarkable photographic documentation of the practice of medicine in the nineteenth century, compiled by Stanley B. Burns, MD, that has been the subject of numerous exhibitions around the world. Among this collection is a stunning history of dermatology through photographs of skin conditions and treatments, many of which have been internationally recognized as photographic masterpieces.

As part of Doak's commitment to the field of dermatology, and the Company's continuing effort to serve physicians and their patients, Doak has commissioned Dr. Stanley Burns and The Burns Archive to produce the first original educational series of four photographic books on the history of dermatology. The images in the collection, sponsored by Doak Dermatologics, were chosen from over 70,000 medical historical photographs in The Burns Archive, many of which have never been seen by the general medical community. These original works will encourage physicians to reflect on the progress of patient treatment. It is interesting to note that many of the same physicians who pioneered the specialty of dermatology also pioneered innovative techniques in the art of medical photography.

Doak is honored to provide this important historical volume because, according to some medical historians, the Company's therapeutic contributions date back to the 1790s. Originally located in Cleveland, Ohio, Doak moved to Westport, NY in 1957. In 1994, Bradley Pharmaceuticals purchased Doak and moved the Company to its current location in Fairfield, NJ.

The purchase by Bradley marked a dramatic rebirth for Doak as it entered the innovative keratolytic market, providing therapies such as the **CARMOL**® **40** line, introduced in 1997, and the **KERALAC**™ line, including **KERALAC**™ (35% Urea) **Lotion** and **KERALAC**™ (50% Urea) **Nail Gel**, introduced in 2004, and **KERALAC**™ (50% Urea) **Cream**, introduced in 2005. Doak also provides acne and rosacea therapies, such as the **ROSULA**® line, including **ROSULA**® (Sodium Sulfacetamide 10% and Sulfur 5% in a Urea vehicle) **Aqueous Gel** and **ROSULA**® (Sodium Sulfacetamide 10% and Sulfur 5% in a Urea vehicle) **Aqueous Cleanser**, both introduced in 2003, and **ROSULA**® **NS** (Sodium Sulfacetamide in a 10% Urea vehicle) **Medicated Pads**, as well as the **ZODERM**® moisturizing benzoyl peroxide product line, both introduced in 2004. In 2004, Doak's parent company, Bradley Pharmaceuticals, through the acquisition of Bioglan Pharmaceuticals Company, obtained **SOLARAZE**® (Diclofenac Sodium-3%) **GEL**, an effective and well-tolerated actinic keratosis treatment, and **ADOXA**® doxycycline tablets for the adjunctive treatment of severe acne. All the preceding important brands have helped build Doak into a multimillion-dollar corporation. Please see full Prescribing Information.

Thank you for your continued support of Doak Dermatologics.

Sincerely,

Daniel Glassman
President and CEO

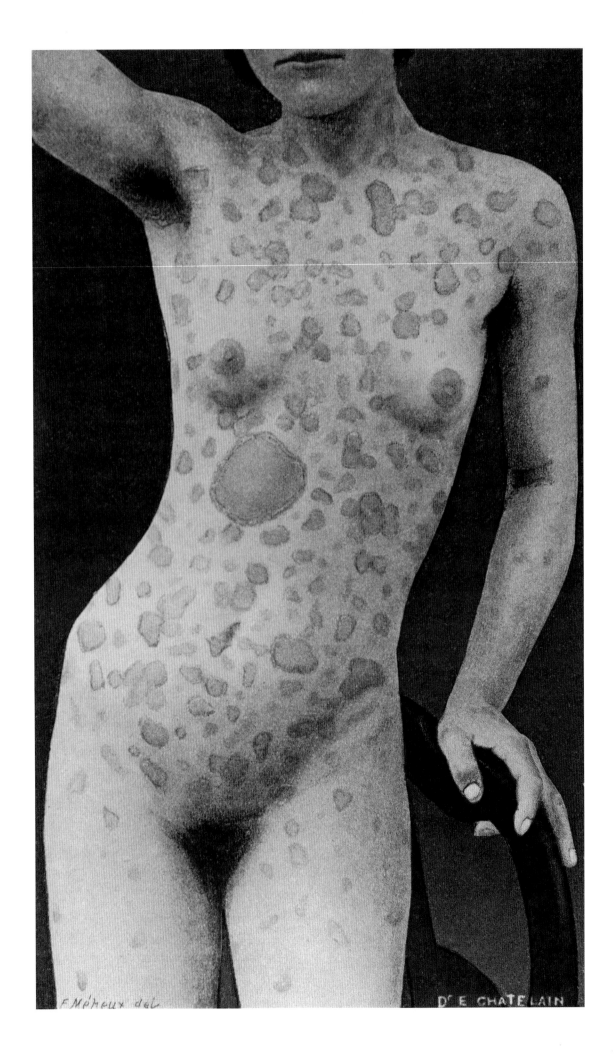

F. Némeux del.   Dʳ E. CHATELAIN

PHOTOGRAPHIC HISTORY OF NINETEENTH CENTURY
DERMATOLOGY
SELECTIONS FROM THE BURNS ARCHIVE

THE TORSO

STANLEY B. BURNS, MD, FACS

BURNS ARCHIVE PRESS
NEW YORK 2005

This first edition of *Photographic History of Nineteenth Century Dermatology, Selections from The Burns Archive: The Torso* is limited to 5,000 copies. The photographs are copyright Stanley B. Burns, MD & The Burns Archive. The text and contents of this volume are copyright Stanley B. Burns, MD, 2005. Printed and bound in China for The Burns Archive Press, NY, a division of Burns Archive Photographic Distributors, Ltd. NY

Care has been taken to confirm the accuracy of the information presented and to describe generally accepted practices. The author has checked with sources believed to be reliable in the effort to provide correct information. New research especially on historical subjects may bring to light new discoveries. The field of medical photographic history is about two decades old. The author would appreciate and encourage readers to write and provide additional or new information and also to add to the iconography.

Copyright © 2005 Stanley B. Burns, MD & The Burns Archive

Published by The Burns Archive Press, an imprint of The Burns Archive,
New York, New York & Germantown, New York

ISBN 0-9748688-7-6

Library of Congress Cataloging-in-Publication Data:
Burns, Stanley B.
Photographic History of Nineteenth Century Dermatology, Selections from The Burns Archive: The Torso
    Includes bibliographical references: 1. Medical, History 2. Dermatology 3. Skin Disease
    4. Psoriasis 5. Syphilis 6. Photography, History 7. Medical, Journals 8. Stanley B. Burns, MD

THE BURNS ARCHIVE PRESS

Author & Publisher:	Stanley B. Burns, MD, FACS
Production & Design:	Elizabeth A. Burns
Editors:	Sara Cleary-Burns & Elizabeth A. Burns
Photographs:	Stanley B. Burns, MD & The Burns Archive

FRONT COVER: PSORIASIS CIRCINATA George Henry Fox, MD, New York, 1900

This image, from *Photographic Atlas of the Diseases of the Skin*, 1900, by George Henry Fox, documents a case of psoriasis circinata. This form of the disease "results from a tendency of the rounded, marginate patches to heal in the centre while the border remains thickened and scaly." This patient had psoriasis for many years, increasing at times then almost disappearing. The lesions leave a geographic-like design on the patient.

FRONTISPIECE: PITYRIASIS ROSEA DE GIBERT E. Chatelain, MD & Félix Méheux, Paris, 1893

In 1860, Parisian dermatologist Camille Melchior Gibert (1797-1866) described a dermatitis with eruptions of small, slightly rosy-colored furfuraceous marks that lasted about 6 to 8 weeks then disappeared without sequellae. During the nineteenth century, numerous dermatologists described and renamed this condition with personal eponyms, among them Bazin, Wilson, Hebra & Kaposi, Vidal, Besnier, and Fournier. However, the original designation 'Pityriasis rosea de Gibert,' survived, and its etiology has been recently agreed upon. At the Congress of the European Academy of Dermatology and Venereology in Barcelona, November 2003, the pityriasis rosea of Gibert (PRG) was decreed, "a spontaneously resolving acute eruption is of herpes viral origin." Most likely, the virus is the HHV6 and/or the HHV7 (Herpes Virus family). No treatment is required. It is a benign affliction prevalent in young adults, especially in the spring. Epidemics can occur, and there is only rare individual recurrence. In 1893, this photograph appeared in *Précis iconographique des maladies de la peau* by Parisian dermatologist E. Chatelain. Félix Méheux, the world-renowned medical photographer and painter at the Hôpital Saint-Louis (1884-1904), took the photographs and his name appears prominently on the front cover. It is the only dermatological photographic atlas to give a cover credit to the photographer. Méheux's artistic painterly abilities are evident in this photograph. William Corlett, MD, professor of dermatology at Cleveland's Western Reserve University School of Medicine, called upon Méheux to paint photographs for his 1901 *Treatise on the Acute Infections Exanthemata*. Méheux painted twelve of Corlett's photographs, highlighting only the diseased areas. He rendered a modernist style of photographic art, now becoming increasingly popular. Unfortunately, the reproductions of Méheux's painted photographs in Chatelain's book are a great visual disappointment. They were reproduced in a variety of chromolithographic-halftones, which are less detailed and realistic than mechanical prints. It is unfortunate that no dermatological work contains Méheux's work as original or mechanical prints. In 1995, noted Parisian dermatologists Daniel Wallach, Jean-Paul Escande and others brought general public awareness to Méheux's images. They showcased Méheux's original dermatological photographs in a museum exhibition and book, *À Corps et à raison, photographies médicales, 1840-1920.*

CONTENTS

DEDICATION

This book is dedicated to New York's George Henry Fox, MD, for his pioneer work in medical photography. He was the most prolific publisher of dermatological photographic works in the nineteenth century, achieving worldwide recognition, as his books were translated into other languages. After serving in the Civil War, Fox studied medicine and began writing and compiling his astounding series of photographic atlases. This was dermatology's pre-therapeutic era, a time of careful observation, detailed descriptions, and hopeful classification of disease. His atlases on dermatology achieved extraordinary success and generations of physicians used them, well into the twentieth century. His work, highlighted in this series, contains some of the most dramatic and artistic visual presentations of skin diseases ever published. It was not only Fox's brilliant visual perception and photographic eye that made the atlases masterpieces; it was also his formidable writing talent. He had the ability to shed the verbosity and pomposity of the era, especially prevalent in medical writing, and present concise, pertinent and essential details of his subject, making his writing memorable. He was also a compassionate writer, whose kindness was evident in the carefully worded descriptions of his diseased patients, stirring a common humanity in his readers. Even now, a century and a quarter later, his atlases are still a lively and, in many instances, accurate read.

During his 91-year life span, Fox was both a major participant in and a witness to the development of the modern profession. He was a founder and president of several dermatological associations, including The American Dermatological Association in 1876. Fox's 1926 autobiographical sketch, *Reminiscences*, creates a window into the personalities and world of late nineteenth century dermatology and dermatologists. Curiously, he devoted only a page and a half to his own publications. By the end of his life, Fox was probably the most admired man to ever practice dermatology. Fox's major nineteenth century publications are: *Photographic Illustrations of Skin Diseases: Non syphilitic* (series of 12 monthly fascicles), 1879; *Photographic Illustrations of Skin Diseases: Non syphilitic*, 1880; *Photographic Illustrations of Cutaneous Syphilis*, 1881; *Illustrated Medicine & Surgery* with Frederick Sturgis, MD, 1884; *Photographic Illustrations of Skin Diseases: Second Edition*, 1885; *Photographic Illustrations of Skin Diseases: Second Edition: Second Series*, 1887 (1888, 1890, 1892); *Illustrated Medicine & Surgery, Second Edition* with F. Sturgis, MD, 1892; "Skin Diseases of Children", *American Journal of Obstetrics* (12 articles), 1896-67; *Skin Diseases of Children*, 1897; *Photographic Atlas of the Diseases of the Skin*, 1900.

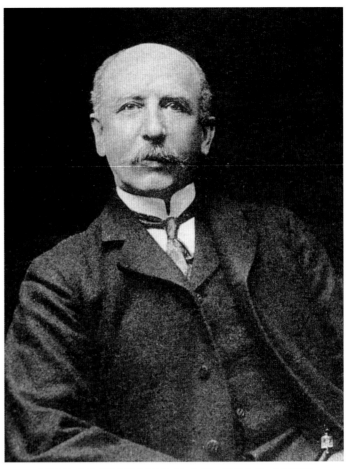

GEORGE HENRY FOX, MD (1846-1937)

After graduating from the Medical College of the University of Pennsylvania in 1869, Fox spent three additional years seeking advanced training at Europe's leading dermatological centers. In 1873, he returned to New York City to set up practice. While working at the Northern Dispensary, he began to photograph interesting patients at a local studio. He put these images on display at the Medical Journal Association's office on East 28th Street, where publisher E.B. Treat admired them and suggested a publication. Fox's atlases were the first medical works to use a new mechanical photographic printing process developed in 1878 called the Artotype, which created a permanent print that did not fade. He also decided to have each photograph hand-painted by Joseph Gaertner, MD, a skilled artist and physician who had studied art and then skin diseases at Vienna's General Hospital (Allegmanes Krankenhaus), the world's leading dermatological institute at that time. Each image was individually painted, so that the colors and painting vary not only from edition to edition but within each volume. In later editions, copy prints of photographs from earlier works were used, resulting in these images being less detailed. Many of the photographs were taken by O.G. Mason, the official in-house photographer for Bellevue Hospital.

Fox held several appointments during his career. He succeeded William H. Draper, MD, as clinical professor of diseases of the skin and chair at the College of Physicians and Surgeons of New York from 1880-1907. He was also chief of the dermatological teaching service of The Skin and Cancer Hospital, a division of the New York Post Graduate Medical School and Hospital from 1883-1913. His son, dermatologist Howard Fox, joined and continued his practice. The preface in Fox's early dermatological atlases has become the classical statement of the importance of photography in dermatology: "The study of Skin Diseases without cases or colored plates is like the study of osteology without bones, or the study of geography without maps. However comprehensive or practical a text-book may be, its verbal descriptions cannot compare in value with a sight of the thing described, or what is next best, its faithful representation. A systematic course of clinical study is only possible in our large cities, and yet the physician in any remote locality may be called upon to treat the rarest forms of skin disease. As success must depend in great measure upon the correctness of his diagnosis, it is hardly necessary to argue the value of a complete series of well-executed plates..."

Fox also contributed to the identification of dermatological disease. In 1888, he described 'match box dermatitis', which is considered the first report on contact dermatitis. In 1902, with John A. Fordyce, MD (1858-1925), he described a rare apocrine sweat gland disease called by the eponym, Fox-Fordyce disease. It is due to a blockage of apocrine sweat glands, which results in chronic itchy patches and is localized to apocrine gland-bearing areas.

In 2004, during my research, I made two significant discoveries that added to the stature of Dr. Fox. The first was finding 12 articles on the skin diseases of children that had been published in the *American Journal of Obstetrics*... They contained 12 beautiful multi-image heliotype plates and over 60 photographs. This was indeed a newly recognized publication, as no prior work mentions its existence. The articles are indicative of Fox's effort to educate physicians in other specialties on dermatological disease. The second discovery occurred at a New York City flea market, where a unique collection of Fox's photographic lantern slides appeared for sale. He used these slides in his lectures. Perhaps further research will result in new discoveries about Fox and his images.

PREFACE

As an ophthalmologist, a life-long collector and a historian, I am fascinated by our past and drawn to visualizing history. When I first started collecting medical photographs in 1975, I chose images based on both their importance as historic documents and as evidence of medicine's rich past. What I soon realized was their artistic strength. In 1979, I created The Burns Archive, which is dedicated to preserving medical photographs and producing publications on the history of medical photography. By the mid-1980s, noted curators and artists became interested in medical photography as art. In 1984, Marvin Heiferman curated "In the Picture of Health," an exhibit of more than 140 photographs from the Archive. This was the first exhibition of medical photographs displayed in a public art institution. In 1987, Joel-Peter Witkin edited *Masterpieces of Medical Photography: Selections from The Burns Archive*. Since then, numerous international major museums and galleries have recognized the artistic value of these images. They now collect and exhibit vintage medical photographs of patients, procedures and practitioners for the general public.

Over the decades, I have learned that art matters. Art elevates and stimulates us to see things differently. Art creates a different perspective and point of view. When medical photographs are presented to the public, the images are viewed and conceived in terms of personal mortality, human fragility and the vagaries of life. Terror and fascination draw the non-medical public into dialogue with these images. Although the art world's appreciation of vintage medical photography as art is laudable, my original goal was to present these photographs to my colleagues not as art, but as historic documents. I wanted my fellow physicians to visually experience the practice of medicine in the nineteenth century to help them gain a better understanding of the foundation of our therapies and patient treatment. As a physician, I am transported back to a different reality by these photographs. I see my patients, I see difficulties in therapy, I see personal challenges and I wonder whether what I am doing and what I believe in will one day be proven wrong. Over the past 150 years our understanding of the nature and especially the etiology of dermatological disease has drastically changed.

This series offers the practitioner a comprehensive collection of significant masterpieces of nineteenth century dermatological photography. It is not meant to be an encyclopedic history of the topic, but rather a compilation emphasizing iconic and artistic photographs that will allow you to see the transition of dermatological medicine from yesterday to today. My hope is that you will look at these images as visual icons of our past and be led to a better understanding of what we do and how we can better serve our patients.

Medicine's quest to unselfishly help and heal is one of mankind's highest goals. I am proud to be part of the profession and to share these photographs to further that goal.

Stanley B. Burns, MD, FACS
New York, June 2005

INTRODUCTION

Photography was a key that enabled dermatologists to unlock the secrets of skin disease. This is the first photographic historical work to document the history of dermatology during its evolution into the modern specialty. This compilation of photographs showcases the patients whom nineteenth century dermatologists encountered while categorizing and naming skin diseases. Photography has served dermatology perhaps more than any other clinical specialty. Invented in the 1830s, it was available as this specialty was developing. Because dermatology is the most visual of the clinical specialties, astute observation of a patient was often the key to diagnosis. Photographs allowed the medical community to share their patients' conditions for the purposes of education and consultation. During the pioneering years of published medical photography - the 1860s and 1870s - dermatologists produced more photographic atlases than did physicians in any other specialty. This series presents photographs from the most noted works. The pictures were primarily chosen for the artistic beauty of early medical imagery. As dermatological disease was often both disfiguring and extensive, pioneer dermatologists and their photographers took great care to present the subject with the highest possible artistic standards while accurately documenting the conditions. These rare photographs are from private albums and sources within The Burns Archive. Many are either published here for the first time or have not been published since their original presentation. In this series of four books, each volume will showcase the disease states of a different of the body: face, torso, extremities and back.

Until the mid-twentieth century, the specialty was officially named "dermatology and syphilology." Dermatologists were usually the first to diagnose and treat syphilis. Syphilis could mimic almost every known disease and would almost always present in some sort of cutaneous lesion. In the nineteenth century, syphilis cases made up about half of a dermatologist's practice. Unfortunately, a good deal of medical photographic history has been lost or destroyed. For one thing, few physicians wished to preserve the evidence of poor treatment or erroneous diagnoses and theories. For another, the pictures were judged too horrific to view. However, many of the images that have survived serve to illustrate the progress and hope of medicine, as most of these conditions are no longer encountered in their advanced states. Fortunately, many dermatological images did survive, since publication of the cutaneous disease photographs for educational purposes was critical to the profession. In addition, some unique albums accumulated by practitioners have been preserved. These photographs provide an unparalleled glimpse through a window of time allowing us to explore the world of our predecessors, their patients and their shared tribulations.

PHOTOGRAPHY IN PUBLICATIONS

This series pays tribute to the physicians who recognized the power of photography to accurately portray dermatological disease and who published the pioneering photographic works: Louis Duhring, Howard F. Dammon, Henry G. Piffard, George Henry Fox, Balmanno Squire, Alfred Hardy, and A. de Montméja. These physicians were instrumental in establishing the modern specialty, producing visual texts that educated hundreds of other practitioners. They took dramatic photographs of their patients, not only so they could share the conditions with their colleagues, but also to document their experiences. This series contains photographs from all of the dermatological atlases of George Henry Fox. Insight into the need for color in dermatological imagery is provided by notable examples of the highly regarded hand-tinted photographs from the dermatological atlases of Parisian Alfred Hardy and London's Balmanno Squire. This series is also the first dermatological publication to present images from both of the pioneer medical photographic journals, Philadelphia's *Photographic Review of Medicine and Surgery* and Paris' *Revue photographique des hôpitaux de Paris*. Photographs from most of the nineteenth century dermatological atlases are represented, as are images documenting skin diseases published by specialists in other fields. Presented for the first time in a dermatological text are photographs from the album of Lyon physician Alexandre Lacassagne. This album represents a direct line of dermatologic interest from Lyon's "*Ecole de l'Antiquaille.*" Lacassagne was the son-in-law of leading dermatologist Joseph Rollet and the father of dermatologist Jean Lacassagne. Over 100 years of family interest in dermatologic subjects may explain the creation and survival of this remarkable collection.

During my extensive research, I examined all sources of nineteenth century dermatological photographs, and chose the best from each available publication or physician's collection. I have used the most significant "original" photograph as the focus of this visual history. Thus, while photographer Félix Méheux's work at the Hôpital Saint-Louis is extensive and magnificent, the reproductions of his photographs in E. Chatelain's 1893 atlas are relatively poor compared to photographs taken by others in that era's photographic atlases. Fortunately, in 1995, French dermatologist and noted historian Daniel Wallach produced a magnificent exhibit and catalogue of Méheux's original photographs. I strongly advise exploration of this work. My research also uncovered images in what I consider an unappreciated work by George Henry Fox and the basis for his *Skin Diseases of Children*. In looking for dermatological photographs and in poring over hundreds of unrelated journals, I discovered in the *American Journal of Obstetrics and Diseases of Women and Children* (1896-97) a dozen articles containing a total of 77 photographs, including beautiful mechanical prints. Some of the images are true icons of the era.

EVOLUTION OF DISEASE

For most of the last 160 years, the practice of medicine has been in a constant state of flux. The nineteenth century developments of general anesthesia, antiseptic/aseptic surgery, the germ theory of disease and the discovery of the X-ray pulled medicine out of its dark age and propelled it into the modern era. Since then almost every generation has seen miraculous changes; diseases once common have become rare, and previously unrecognized or new diseases have come to the forefront of concern. In the era covered in this series, tuberculosis was the number one killer in developed countries and syphilis was a scourge that threatened not only individuals but also the very foundations of society.

In an era in which few specific efficacious therapies existed and surgical treatment was often equated with death, patients allowed diseases, many now conquered, to develop to extremes. As physicians sought answers to help their patients, they photographed the conditions that most concerned them. This series depicts many of those images. Also documented are some rare instances where therapy was evaluated. To reflect the ideology of the era, many of the photographs are accompanied by the comments of the physicians or other experts of the period. With the advantage of 20/20 hindsight, the modern physician will be able to understand what the period physician was thinking and how modern dermatology has clarified some important theories. These texts accurately capture the incomplete state of knowledge of the time; indeed, some offer insight to accurate portrayal of disease states against the mainstream concepts of the era. One example is Dr. David Gruby's identification of the cause of fungal skin diseases in the 1840s, some 40 years before the germ theory of disease.

PHOTOGRAPHIC ICONOGRAPHY OF DERMATOLOGY

This series not only creates a masterwork of pioneer dermatological photography, it presents a valuable new historic entity for the profession. It offers an iconography of dermatological publications with original photographs. The series and iconography end at the beginning of the twentieth century (1901) because by then, the half-tone photograph, created by grids, had become commonplace and had replaced mechanical prints. Photographs in textbooks and atlases then became mass-produced, with poorer quality reproductions. This iconography is a clear starting point for bibliophiles and historians to study the development of dermatological photography and hopefully to add to the list of dermatological images.

PHOTOGRAPHS AS DERMATOLOGICAL ART & HISTORICAL DOCUMENTS

I am concerned with the primacy of the photograph as opposed to the photographer. The photographs are the power and emphasis of this historic series, and they were chosen with the idea of creating a work of contextual masterpieces of dermatological images. The strength of these historic photographs as art and medicine is to inform, teach and create empathy and appreciation for our predecessors' trials and tribulations. Many of these photographs were taken as calls for help, perhaps not only within the period, but also in terms of future analysis. Photographs helped to rewrite medical history, as many of the diseases described as one entity were ultimately found to be another. Photographs crystallize the link between the observed diseases, providing a permanent memento for both current and future analysis. It is my hope that the reader will be engaged by the photographs and gain a better understanding of the nature of the practice of medicine. Because most people think visually, photographs provide keys to remembrance, enhancing our comprehension and education. Iconic photographs and stories are indelibly etched into our conscience. This collection of powerful images includes examples of masterpieces of medical photography and the art and mystique of medicine. The descriptive text highlights the medical accomplishments and their pertinent photographic historical relevance. This astonishing compilation of images stands as a testament to the effort of health care practitioners to heal and comfort. The photographs not only reveal the challenges met by our predecessors, but provide visual tools with which modern practitioners may contemplate their own work and appreciate their role in the history of this profession.

THE TORSO - VOLUME 2

Faces generally are not hidden from view, while the bulk of the body, with the exception of the hands, can be well disguised. Severe cases of syphilis and other maladies could usually be concealed. Shame, modesty and fear of treatment encouraged patients to ignore their disease until it progressed to the extreme. Shown in this series are both common and uncommon skin diseases. Taking their cues from the art world, photographers posed and lit their subjects as artistically as possible, since in most cases patients were photographed in the nude. Acknowledged in this volume is the monumental contribution by New York dermatologist George Henry Fox, MD, in the promotion of dermatological photography. He was the most prolific dermatological photographic publisher, and images from his various books from 1879 through 1900 are presented. Photographs from a recently discovered, unappreciated work by Fox, *Skin Diseases of Children*, will appear throughout the series. These photographs have not been reproduced since their original presentation and some of the images are truly iconic, visually summing up the entire era.

I

CONGENITAL ICHTHYOSIS Alexandre Lacassagne, MD, Lyon, circa 1895

This image is part of a series taken by Alexandre Lacassagne, MD (1843-1924), of a patient with congenital ichthyosis. This disorder of cornification of the skin is characterized by hyperkeratosis or 'scaling.' In 1902, Jean-Louis Brocq, MD (1856-1928), defined the varieties of ichthyosis, naming the condition "congenital ichthyosiform erythroderma," a term derived from the 'fish-scale' appearance of the skin. Today, the disease is differentiated into several variants. In the rare bullous form, epidermolytic hyperkeratosis, the patient is born with raw, tender skin and the condition is usually lifelong. The more common form, ichthyosis vulgaris, is probably what this patient suffered. In most cases, the scaly areas are small and isolated with symptoms occurring gradually in early childhood. Over time, the typical cornification hardens the skin and creates a reptilian scale-like covering over the affected areas and often disappears during adulthood. Both of these types of ichthyosis are inherited as autosomal dominant traits. There is a series of acquired disorders of cornification related to immune, metabolic, neoplastic, and nutritional diseases and medications.

Ichthyosis is considered one of the most visually fascinating deformities and "alligator-skinned or fish-skinned" people were often seen in sideshows. In the nineteenth century, people with congenital deformities, unusual injuries or other physical maladies could earn a living displaying their conditions or selling photographs of themselves. It was a respectable living and some of them, such as Siamese twins Cheng & Eng and Millie & Sissy, became quite rich. Physicians often reported the cases they encountered at sideshows. Dermatologist George Henry Fox reports several cases in his series of *Photographic Illustrations of Skin Diseases*:

Dr. L. P. Yandell has reported (*Louisville Med. News*, 1878) an interesting case of ichthyosis, which was on public exhibition as the "Man-fish of Tennessee." He presents a magnificent example of the form of the disease which has been called Ichthyosis serpentina, the resemblance of his skin to the skin of a boa-constrictor being almost perfect. About his joints the skin was loose and wrinkled. Upon the belly and limbs the scales were large and suggestive of the skin of a lizard or alligator. The cuticle was everywhere dry and hard and there was no perspiration. The man was fifty years of age, but being shrunken and withered he appeared like a very old man. The skin of the face was red and shining and tightly drawn about the cheeks, pulling the lower lids down to such an extent as to perfectly evert them and making a horrid case of Ectropion. The fingers and toes seemed shorter than natural and the separation between them extended much further down then usual suggesting a webbed condition. He was the father of several children, none of whom inherited the disease.

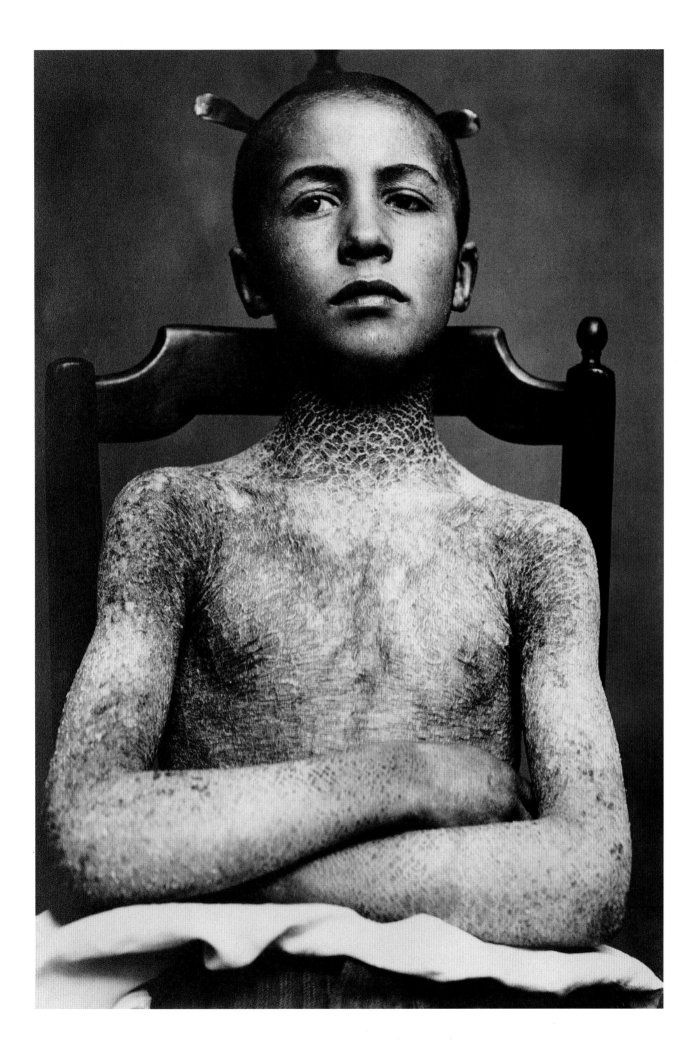

SYPHILIDE VESICULEUSE Alfred Hardy, MD & A. de Montméja, MD, Paris, 1868

The dermatological atlas *Clinique photographique de l'hôpital Saint-Louis*, published by Alfred Hardy and A. de Montméja in 1868, contained some of the most artistically posed and painted photographs of early medical photography. This image of vesicular syphilis has been republished and exhibited numerous times. Of the 50 photographs in the atlas, this is one of five that has received widespread acclaim. The image is an icon of an age when syphilis ruled as the captain of all venereal diseases, but was at times overlooked by amorous suitors. The beauty of the woman and mild expression of her deadly disease is in contrast with most cases of cutaneous syphilis (see number 7). Hardy describes the varieties of skin lesions associated with vesicular cutaneous syphilis. He uses the term 'variola,' which is the name modern medicine associates with smallpox. However, the discrete vesicular lesion of syphilis was typically called by this term. As a result, in nineteenth century dermatological case histories, the term "varioloid" or "variola" describing a rash seems like a polite word to describe syphilis. Smallpox was always a concern and Hardy explains the differentiation from a mild case of smallpox in his description of vesicular syphilis:

Syphilis rarely manifests in this form of an eruption. We distinguish between three types of vesicular syphilis: the variola form, the eczematous and the herpetiforme.The variola form appears four to six months after the initial incident. It is characterized by red marks which can reach the size of a pea. On these marks one or two transparent elevated vesicles can form which are globular or umbilicated with a central depression. The content of the vesicles pours out when they rupture and can form an adherent crust with a typical syphilitic color. The areola that surrounds the lesion demonstrates the same general color. At the end of ten to twenty days the projection collapses leaving a small macule which will not disappear for a while. This type of eruption repeats successively for several months and most of the time in the same region. The vesicles are generally isolated and very rarely confluent (see photograph). Their number is always fairly limited. It is not rare to see on the same individual different phases of evolution of the vesicles, as well as the existence of other skin diseases in the secondary syphilitic class. This variety cannot be confused with any other manifestation of cutaneous syphilis or with any other simple variola because the predromal recurrent fevers are not encountered in other types of syphilis. And the variola (smallpox) reaction manifests in a more rapid eruption along with a rose-colored vesiculopustular lesion, which does not at all resemble the slow eruption of the syphilitic eruption whose red marks are furthermore surrounded by a characteristic halo… Syphilis vesiculose eczematous form differs from the preceding in that the eruption begins with discrete or confluent vesicles surrounded by a reddish-brown ring. When they are aggregated one sees only a dark red surface covered in transparent vesicles larger than those seen in eczema… Syphilis vesiculeuse herpetiforme develops as very small vesicles the size of a grain of millet with a copper colored base and are grouped either irregularly, in rings or concentric circles. The vesicles are more resistant than those found in herpes…

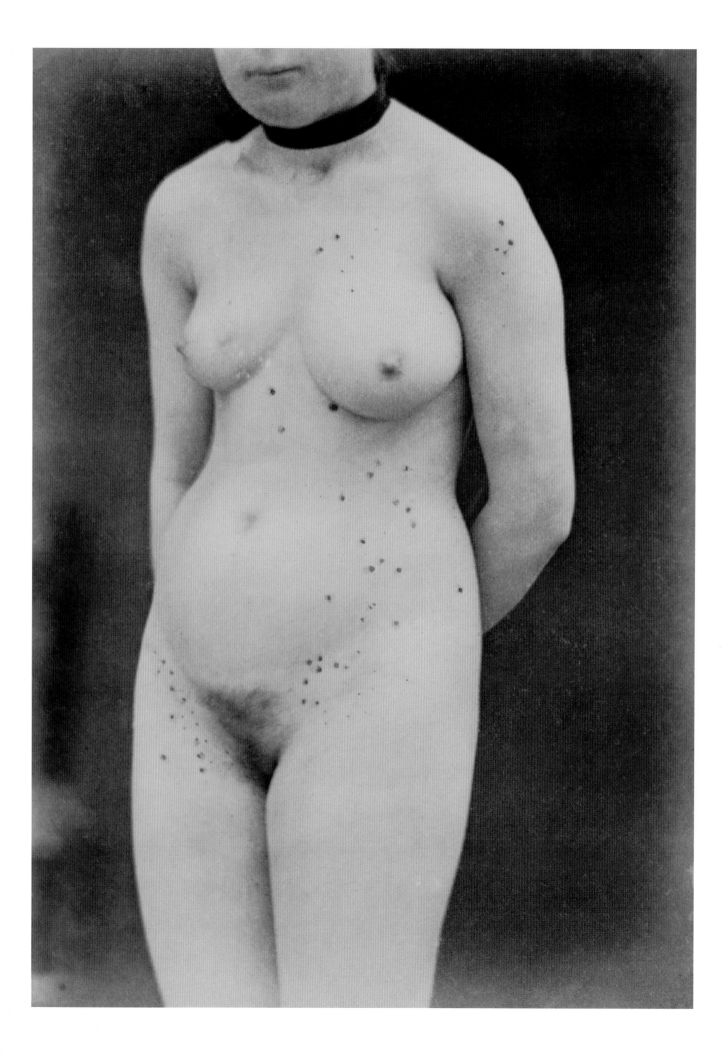

PSORIASIS DIFFUSA George Henry Fox, MD, New York, 1885

George Henry Fox published this image in 1885, in his second edition of *Photographic Illustrations of Skin Disease*. In this atlas, he illustrated various phases of this common disease as well as the latest treatment. His description reads as follows:

> This very common affection consists in circumscribed patches of red and thickened skin, covered usually with whitish or yellowish-white scales. The patches may be isolated or confluent… In the latter case they give rise to large irregular patches, with scalloped borders, and frequently with enclosed areas of normal or slightly pigmented skin. The treatment of a case of psoriasis is simple as far as regards the removal of the eruption. It's a much more difficult matter to prevent its return… Local applications will restore the skin to its normal state in nearly all cases… Patient of L. D. Buckley, MD: In this case the scales had been removed leaving smooth, red, infiltrated patches with an elevated border. Upon the forehead the eruption is seen in a characteristic location.

After removal of the scales, Fox recommends the importance of daily baths, various lotions such as carbolic acid in glycerin or tar as oil of cade. If the scales are hard and difficult to remove, scaling and use of chrysophanic acid in the form of 'chrysarobin' paste used in a variety of dressings is the treatment of choice.

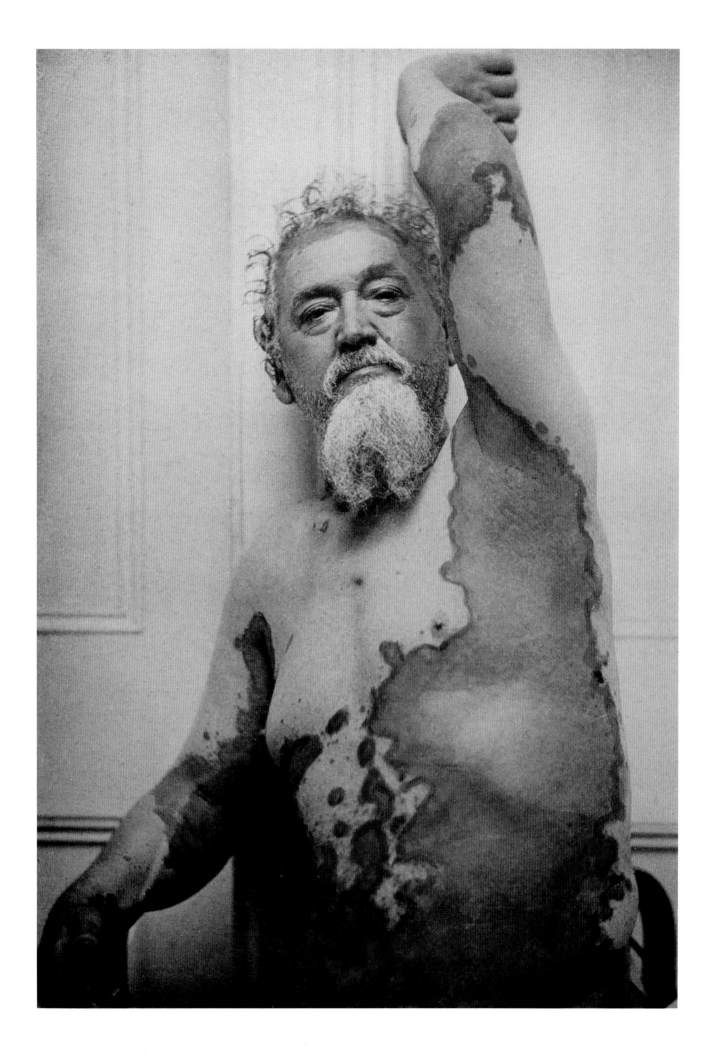

ERYTHEMA ANNULATUM Henry G. Piffard, MD, New York, 1891

Disease often decorates the body with strange and wonderful patterns. Although this young woman appears to be wearing a paisley dress, she is actually experiencing a hypersensitive skin reaction noted as 'erythema annulatum.' This condition is a relatively mild allergic dermal reaction, which has spread over the patient's entire body. Erythema, a hyperemia of the skin, is the first and most common skin reaction caused by an internal or external irritant. Irritants include foods, drugs, chemicals, animals, bacterial or viral substances, as well as radiation, heat or cold, rheumatic fever, insect bites, cancer and sensitivity to one's own tissue. Even psychological disturbances may manifest themselves this way. Treatment for the condition usually and most simply consists of removing the offending causative material.

This photograph was published in 1891 as plate 42 in *A Practical Treatise on Diseases of the Skin* by Henry Granger Piffard, MD (1842-1910). He was Professor of Diseases of the Skin at The University of the City of New York and a pioneer dermatologist responsible for numerous innovations. In May of 1869, he co-founded the New York Dermatological Society, now the oldest dermatological society in the world, and in 1875 created the first postgraduate course in dermatology in North America. In 1876, he wrote the first 'modern' dermatological text in the United States. In 1882, Piffard, with Prince Morrow, MD, started the *Journal of Cutaneous and Venereal Disease*, which evolved into the current *Archives of Dermatology*. Piffard, also an innovator in photography, pioneered indoor photography using a magnesium flash. He was active in photographic organizations and was published in several journals. He took all the photographs for his 1891 atlas using his flash technique. He stated in the preface, "The photographs from which the Plates were prepared were made by the author with the aid of artificial light, which his experience leads him to prefer for this purpose to ordinary light." This book was also the first dermatological atlas produced with a full-page photographic format.

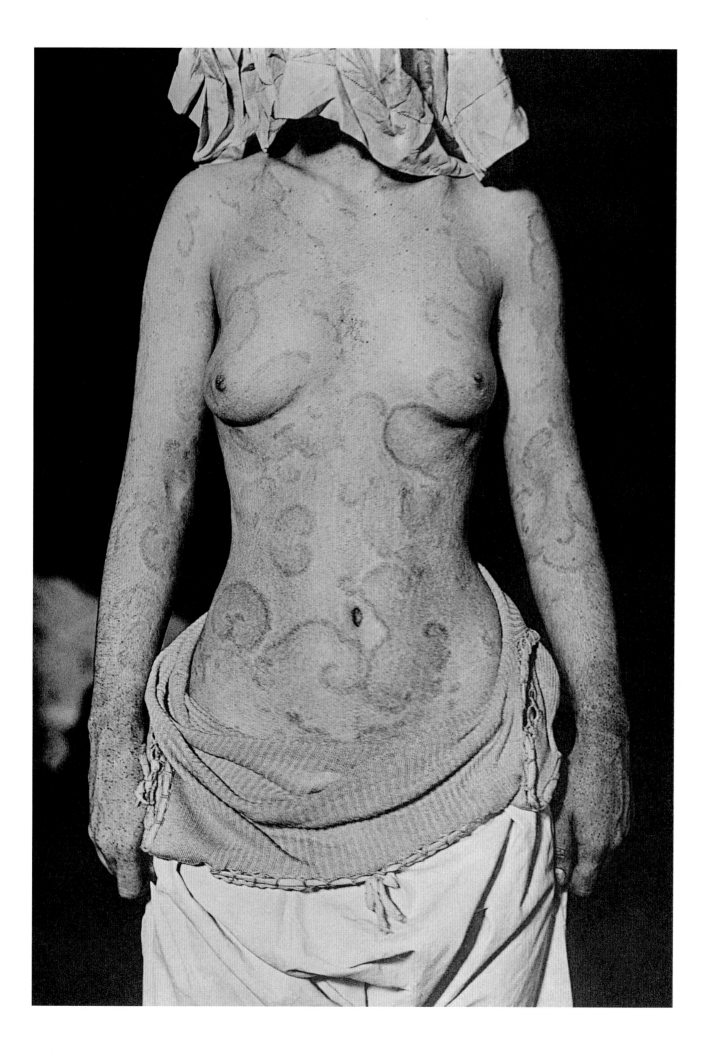

DERMATOGRAPHISM Philadelphia, 1899

This photograph, taken by Philadelphia photographers Gilbert & Bacon, displays a man with "Dermatographism 1899" written on his chest. It was produced as a cabinet card, which is a 4 by 5 1/2 inch photograph mounted on a 4 1/4 by 6 1/2 inch card. These cabinet cards were a standard popular size from 1866 until the end of the first decade of the twentieth century. Physicians would send their patients to photographers and have images taken. Several institutions have collections of cabinet cards albums, some from private collections made by physicians of their own patients, and others from cards sent for consultations. This image was the sole survivor a physician's collection. It was saved because of its uniqueness as a curiosity; the rest were destroyed. Medical photographs were frequently destroyed, but not because of patient concerns. After the death of the physician, heirs simply discarded the images, as they were too disturbing. Fortunately, some physicians donated their collections to institutions that preserved them. Even then, preservation seemed more a matter of luck rather than choice as many institutions discarded or destroyed their collections of old medical photographs.

Skin writing, or dermatographism, is one of the most interesting and bizarre of medical phenomena. It occurs when the skin is touched in states of hypersensitivity. Pressure on the skin results in a localized, temporary raised area of swelling. To document this phenomenon, this patient had his diagnosis and the year written across his chest by his physicians. Today, we know that almost any immunologic, chemical or physical insult can induce the condition. Food allergies are the most common immunologic cause.

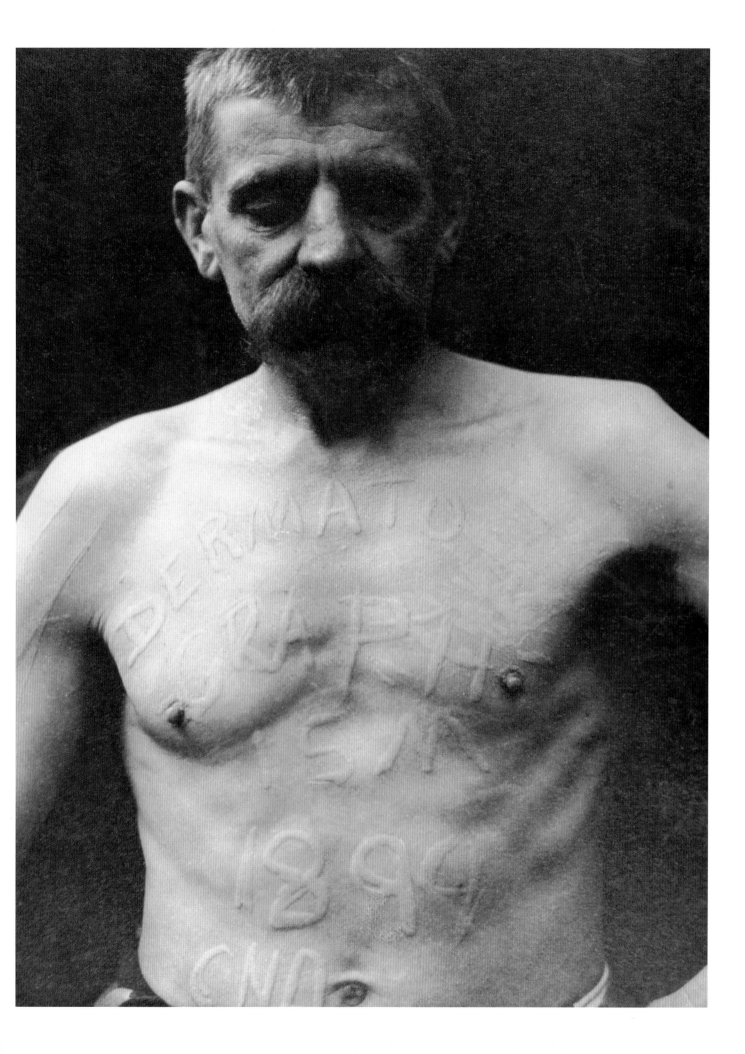

DERMATITIS EXFOLIATIVA George Henry Fox, MD, New York, 1900

This photograph of dermatitis exfoliativa is from George Henry Fox's 1900 *Photographic Atlas of the Diseases of the Skin*. The patient and her potentially fatal condition are described by Fox:

> Dermatitis exfoliativa is used by some writers as a synonym of pityriasis rubra (of Hebra). A distinction should be made, however, since the former disease runs an acute course in many cases and is always amenable to treatment, while the latter disease, although it may begin as an exfoliativa dermatitis, tends to grow worse in spite of treatment and finally results in a smooth, reddened, atrophied skin and terminates fatally. The scaling in this disease is peculiar, the epidermis peeling in large papery flakes. These often curl at the free borders while remaining attached in the centre to the subjacent skin. There is never any moisture of the surface as in eczema, nor any accumulation of silvery epidermic masses as in psoriasis. In exceptional cases a few bullae may develop upon the surface and the eruption bear a strong resemblance to pemphigus foliaceus. The patient, whose trunk and arms are well portrayed in the plate, was sent to the Skin and Cancer Hospital by Dr. Martin Burke. The eruption had developed rapidly and involved the entire body in a few weeks. Under the administration of alkaline diuretics the redness of the skin faded, the scaling gradually lessened, and in two months she left the hospital with an almost normal skin.

'Exfoliativa dermatitis' is now recognized as a common clinical expression of multiple skin disorders. It can be caused by a drug reaction or infection. It is characterized by scaling, itching, hair loss and redness. It is called various names depending on the appearance and/or the cause of the condition. Among the many names now used are erythroderma, scalded skin syndrome, acute toxic epidermolysis, Lyell syndrome, Ritter disease, toxic epidermal necrolysis and others.

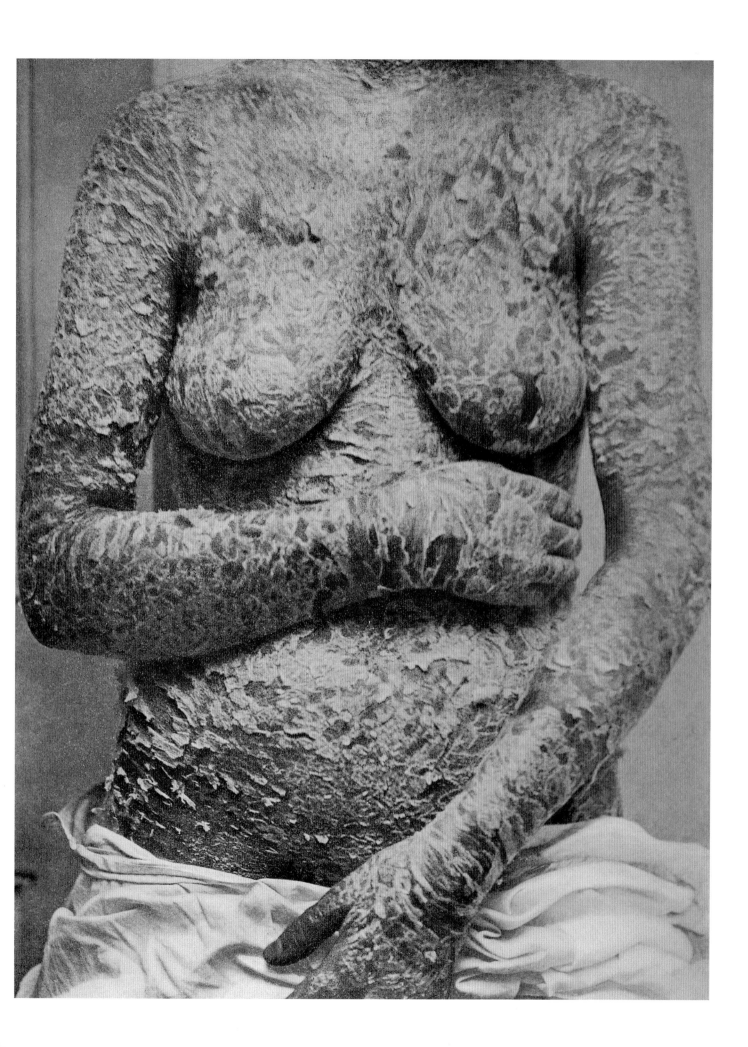

GENERAL TERTIARY SYPHILIS Alexandre Lacassagne, MD, Lyon, circa 1895

This photograph from the album of Alexandre Lacassagne documents a woman with 'generalized tertiary syphilis' and is symbolic of the intensity with which the French studied this disease. Syphilodermas, the cutaneous manifestations of syphilis, most often occurred with similar lesions at each stage; however, when the type of lesions varied, it took an astute dermatologist to suspect and identify the disease. The late syphilitic eruptions were unsymmetrical, as seen here, and consisted of more invasive lesions such as gummas, tubercles, ulcers and pustulo-crustaceous lesions.

Throughout most of the nineteenth century, the French led the world in understanding, teaching and expressing the social concerns inherent with venereal disease. In 1838, Philippe Ricord, MD (1800-1899), published *Traité practique des maladies vénériennes*. In this landmark work, Ricord defined the chancre as the initial lesion in syphilis and clearly demonstrated that gonorrhea and syphilis were two distinct diseases. He also divided syphilis into three stages - primary, secondary and tertiary. Others followed Ricord in clarifying and separating syphilis from other diseases. In 1852, Léon Bassereau, MD (1811-1888), described the separateness of soft chancre (chancroid) from the syphilitic chancre. In 1876, Jean-Alfred Fournier, MD (1832-1914), identified the syphilitic origin of tabes dorsalis, and, in 1879, the syphilitic origin of the general paralysis of the insane. In 1886, his text on (congenital) hereditary syphilis was published and he became the leader in social concerns of the spread of the disease and in its cultural significance. In 1859, syphilologist/dermatologist Joseph Rollet (1824-1894) of Lyon confirmed the duality of the soft and hard chancre and also demonstrated the contagiousness of secondary syphilis. One of his most important contributions was the clear establishment that multiple venereal diseases could exist in the same person, hence the confusion that there was with chancre, chancroid, gonorrhea and others. 'Rollet's Disease' was the presence of both types of lesions, soft and hard chancres, signifying the presence of multiple venereal diseases.

The Lyon school of venerology and dermatology, created in 1837, was called "de l'Antiquaille." Rollet was its most distinguished leader between 1855 and 1864. He was also the father-in-law of Alexandre Lacassagne, who created this exceptional album. This image and the other photographs from the Lyon album represent a direct line of dermatologic interest from the École de l'Antiquaille. Rollet's grandson, Jean Lacassagne (1886-1960) also practiced dermatology in Lyon. Over 100 years of family interest in dermatological subjects may explain the production of this unique album.

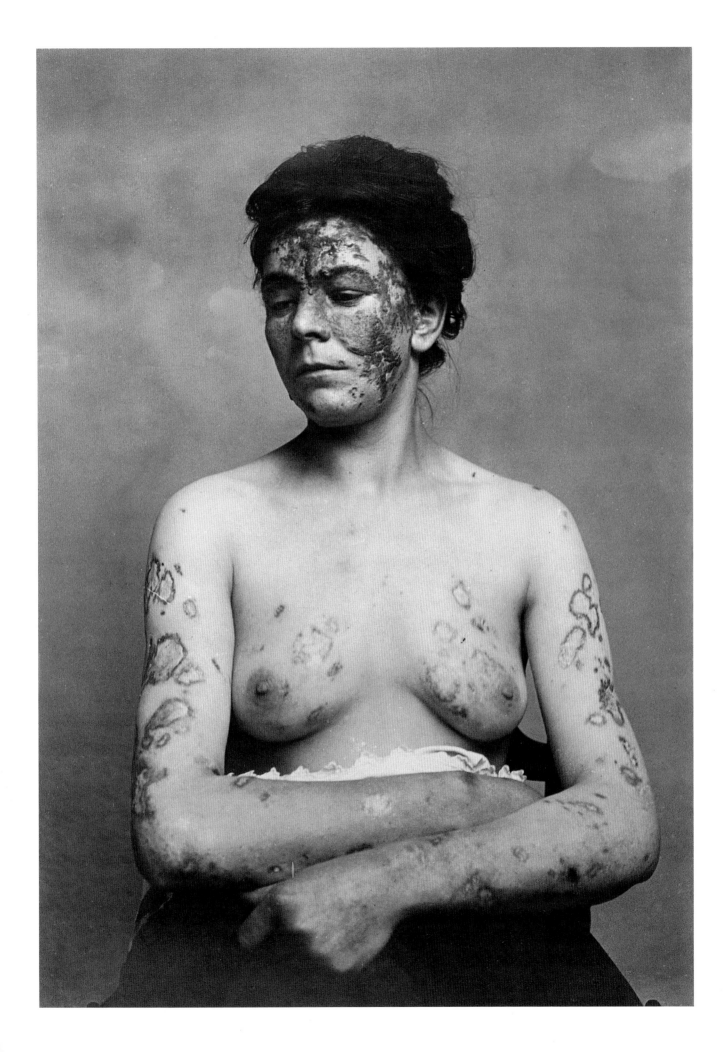

CRIMINAL TATTOOS Alexandre Lacassagne, MD, Lyon, circa 1895

In 1881, Alexandre Lacassagne, MD (1843-1924), published his masterwork, *Les Tatouages, etude anthropologique et médico legale*, on the meaning of tattoos in society, focusing on their implications and associations with criminality. His book and life's work laid the groundwork for later researchers and stimulated generations of proponents in these beliefs. Today, the Lacassagne Institute in Lyon continues his vision and work. This photograph documents the typical wording, as well as images of women, often associated with former prisoners. It was part of a series Lacassagne accumulated of tattooed and dermatological patients, as a research and educational resource. His interest in the markings, designs and pathology of dermatological disease may have been part of the foundation for his study of skin decorations. Lacassagne's father-in-law was the noted dermatologist, Joseph Rollet.

During the nineteenth century, phrenology and physiognomy influenced the ideologies of the medical and scientific communities. At the beginning of the century, phrenology, the study of lumps and bumps on the skull, relating them to personality, behavior and disease, was the most important conceptual psychiatric ideology. It maintained its influence on many until the last decades of the century. Physiognomy, the study of facial features and their relationship to personality and character, had been used as an analytical tool for centuries. In 1872, Charles Darwin's book, *The Expression of the Emotions in Man and Animals*, expanded the field. Darwin showed that certain human expressions were universal and perhaps existed in the animal world. Lacassagne proposed that a tattoo, readable on the skin, served as a visual representation and expression of that person's individuality, but more importantly indicated a group association. In the nineteenth century, tattooing was primarily an art associated with sailors, who picked up the practice from South Sea Island natives. By mid-century it had spread to a lower-class 'criminal' element. Lacassagne attempted to correlate the types, positions, style, depictions and wordings of tattoos to various aspects of criminality. Criminal anthropologists, such as Italian psychiatrist Césare Lombroso, MD (1835-1909), seized upon any visual marker to help identify criminals and incorporated the information into a system of criminal identification. In 1888, his *L'Homme Criminel* expanded Lacassagne's theories.

While tattooing has entered mainstream American culture in the last few decades, it is still used by street gangs and prisoners. Its most noted use can be seen on criminals in the Russian penal system. Now dermatologists often find themselves involved in the treatment of allergic reactions to the pigments and more importantly, in the removal of unwanted tattoos.

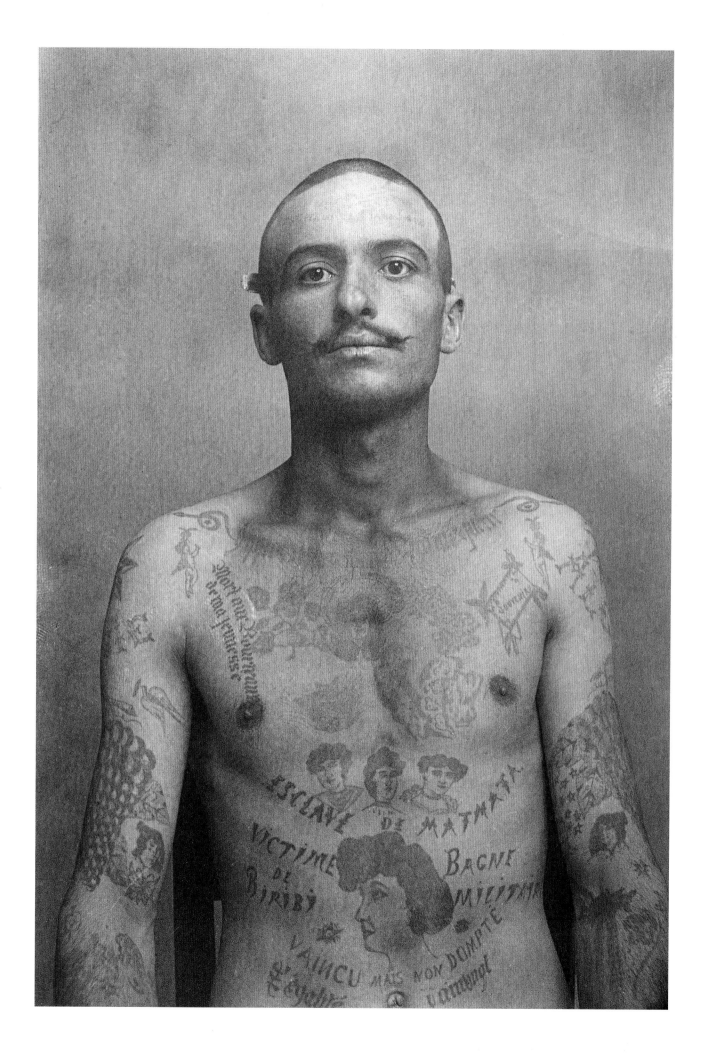

MYCOSIS FUNGOIDES Alexandre Lacassagne, MD, Lyon, circa 1895

In the nineteenth century, the skin manifestations of chronic infectious disease offered such a wide range of expressions that they often mimicked each other. Many patients sought care only when their disease was quite far advanced. To complicate diagnosis, secondary infections with ulcerations in advanced cutaneous disease could create similar appearances. (see *Back,* number 13) This photograph, from an album of dermatological conditions by Lyon physician Alexandre Lacassagne, is one of the only images of massive skin involvement so complex that the experts could not agree on a primary diagnosis. The differentials offered were infected cutaneous syphilis, cutaneous tuberculosis and mycosis fungoides. The disease involved almost one entire side of the torso with a sheet-like covering of deranged tissue in various stages of activity. The groin was the most active area with ulcers, nodules, tubercles, papules and gummatous type lesions. From the groin the lesions decreased in aggressiveness until they ended in a large drape (patches/plaques) that looked like scar tissue. Today, pathological biopsy, bacteriological, hematologic or other laboratory studies could make the diagnosis. Mycosis fungoides is now recognized as part of the cutaneous T-cell lymphoma spectrum. The typical large patches and plaques in this disease appear to be the dominant cutaneous changes suffered by this patient.

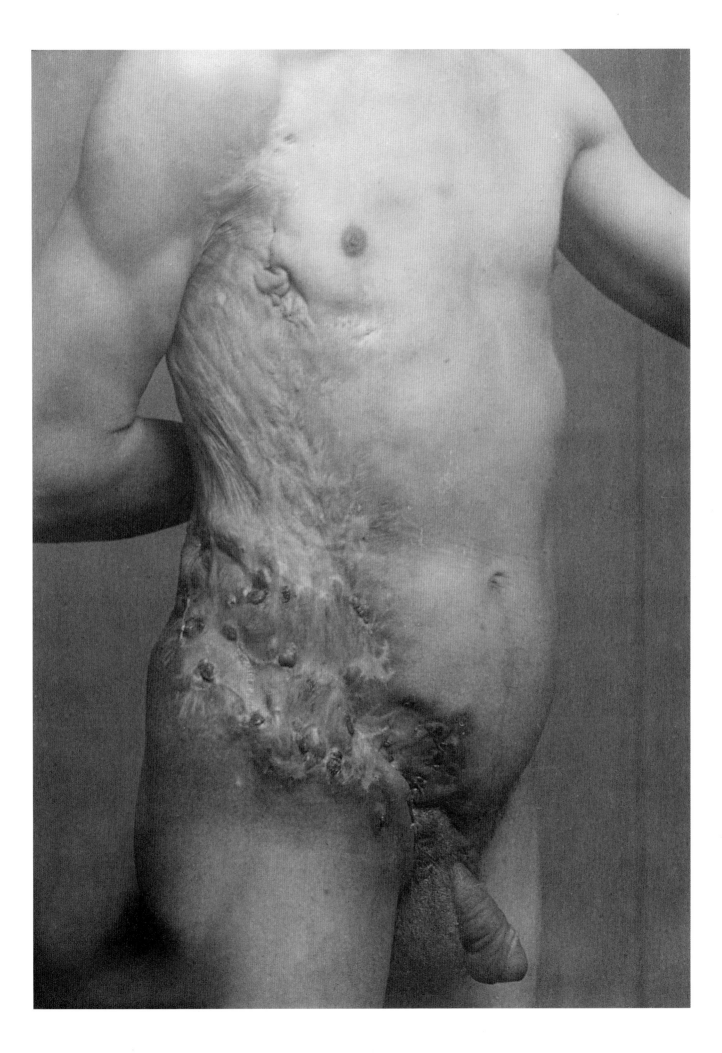

MELASMA IN PHTHEIRIASIS Henry G. Piffard, MD, New York, 1891

This photograph documents an unusual symptom, darkening of the skin, or 'melasma,' caused by a long-term infestation of body lice. In 1891, Henry G. Piffard published this image, taken using his flash technique, in *A Practical Treatise on Diseases of the Skin*. He described the condition in its various forms:

Phtheiriasis is the name applied to the affections produced by the invasion of the three well-known varieties of *pediculus* - namely, the head-louse, body-louse, and pubic or crab louse. The nature and appearance of these insects are so well-known… The first of these infect the scalp; the second confines itself to the non-hairy portions of the surface; and the third prefer the pubic region, but may be met with wherever the hairs are short. Phtheiriasis Capitis: This affection occurs most frequently in children, more rarely in women, and almost never in men… They derive their nourishment from the skin, and by their presence produce considerable itching and lead to a corresponding amount of scratching. In children predisposing to eczema they not infrequently lead to the development of this affection. The diagnosis is, of course readily made, as inspection of the scalp will quickly reveal the presence of the insects and their ova, if at all abundant. In doubtful cases the fine-tooth comb will be found an efficient 'trap'… Phtheiriasis Corporis: the affection is very rarely met with in young persons, and is found most frequently in middle and advanced life, and especially in the feeble and ill-fed, and among the frequenters of prisons and cheap lodgings. Though sometimes met with in women, nine tenths of the cases that come under observation are among men. The *pediculus corpus* does not lodge upon the body, but infests and breeds among the folds of under-garments, from which hiding-places it sallies forth to seek its nourishment… These insects excite a lively and, at times, most atrocious itching, and lead to vigorous scratching… in severe cases extensive excoriations, pustules, and even ulcers. In cases that have lasted for any length of time, the skin gradually darkens, even to the color of a mulatto. (see photograph). Treatment- Soap, water and clean clothes are all that is necessary. Phtheiriasis Pubis: The pediculus pubis affects a preference for the pubic region of both sexes, but is not confined to this locality, but in women may also be met with in the axillary region and in the eyebrows, and in men among the chest-hairs and in the beard and whiskers… The treatment… involves the employment of some anti-parasitic application, and the one most in vogue is the common 'blue-ointment.'

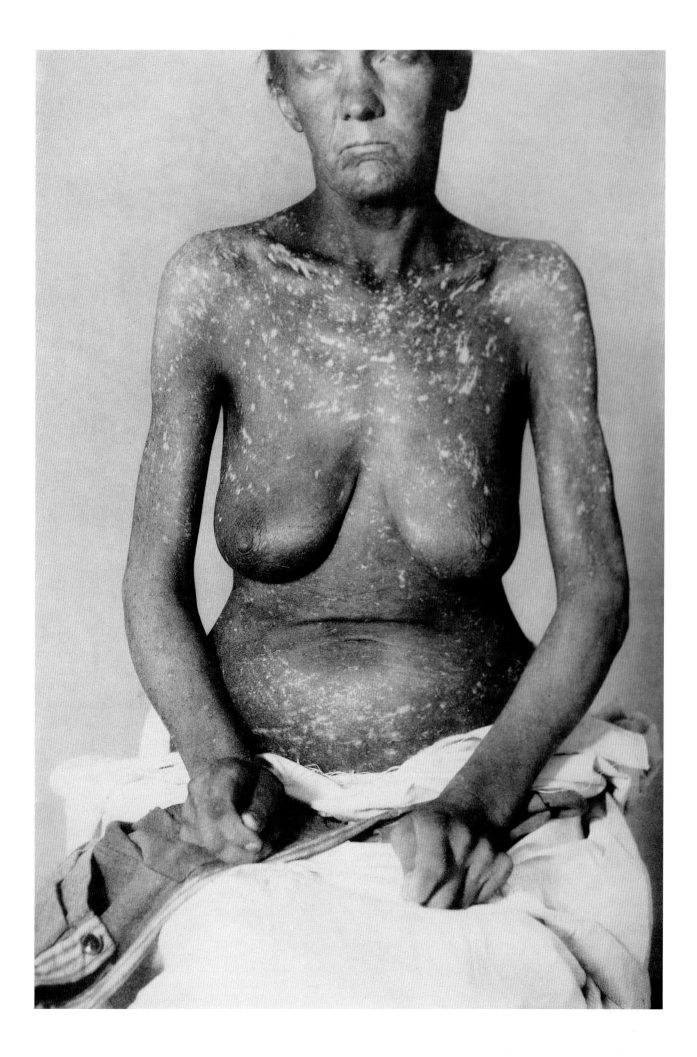

MOLLUSCUM PENDULUM A. de Montméja, MD, Paris, 1869

This photograph of molluscum pendulum appeared in the first issue, 1869, of *Revue photographique des hôpitaux de Paris*. Capturing an image of an extreme disease state was one of Dr. de Montméja's goals and he was certainly successful in this instance. In this era, when a disease was presented in its most severe manifestation, the patient was usually beyond help. However, this particular condition was an exception, as the same level of cure was possible whether the disease was treated early or in an advanced state. The treatment was surgery and involved cutting and then cauterization or ligation of the pedicle. Postoperative infection was a major complication of surgery and any size wound could swiftly become fatal. In 1867, the antiseptic surgical method was described by England's Joseph Lister (1827-1912). When this patient was to be operated on in 1869, only two years after the discovery, anti-sepsis had not been generally accepted and was not the norm until the mid-1880s. The French were among the last to generally adopt the procedure, although some surgeons used it in the 1870s. Pedicle-based lesions offered one of the more satisfactory procedural outcomes.

A fibroma was considered a benign tumor that needed only a simple excision. By 1900, they were recognized as "connective tissue new growth, characterized by the appearance in the skin of flat or pedunculated, rounded, painless, soft or firm tumors of varying size." Molluscum pendulum was an unusual variety, and the condition was described fairly accurately in the 1869 journal. However, terminology has changed and 'molluscum' is now associated mainly with molluscum contagiosum, a benign self-limiting papular eruption of multiple umbilicated cutaneous tumor like lesions caused by a large DNA poxvirus. The disease was first described, in 1817, by English dermatologist Thomas Bateman (1778-1821). The anatomical similarity of multiple fibromas and the multiple small lesions of the viral disease most likely led to the 'molluscum' designation by physicians who diagnosed the diseases by anatomic appearance. By the mid-twentieth century more accurate pathological and laboratory based studies helped to create the modern scientific nomenclature of dermatology. Montméja's journal notes:

The molluscums are a class of fibroma characterized by tubercles spread over the body principally on the neck the perineum and the trunk. This tumor was on the (upper) thigh of a 66 year-old woman. It appeared when she was thirteen; the woman had 17 children but never considered removing the tumor. She finally decided to do so and the operation was performed at the Hôpital Saint-Louis with a 'serre-noeud', that easily detached the tumor without any hemorrhaging. Towards the end, the rubbing of the tumor against the woman's clothing caused two ulcerations which are shown in the photograph. (There are two varieties of molluscum). The first variety, molluscum simplex, falls entirely within the category of skin maladies by the development of multiple tubercle like tumors of various dimensions in localized areas of the body (see number 16). The second variety, molluscum pendulum, by its slow development, and its often-excessive growth, falls entirely within the category of 'tumors'. Venous vessels are apparent on the tumor and give it a purplish color. Sometimes there is oozing, and redness on the surface of the tumor as in our example; this indicates foremost that the molluscum is undergoing an inflammatory period. Drs. Heylaud and (Rudolph) Virchow as well as (August) Nélaton stated that during this type of tumor's course of development, there were inflammatory surges, periods of pain analogous to those appearing with elephantiasis. Also as this tumor has been called, based on a common agreement in France and abroad, molluscum éléphantiasique. The most certain method for removal is the metallic 'serre-noeud,' which destroys the pedicle by obliterating the venous and sometimes fairly large arterial vesicles that it contains (a type of clamp instrument).

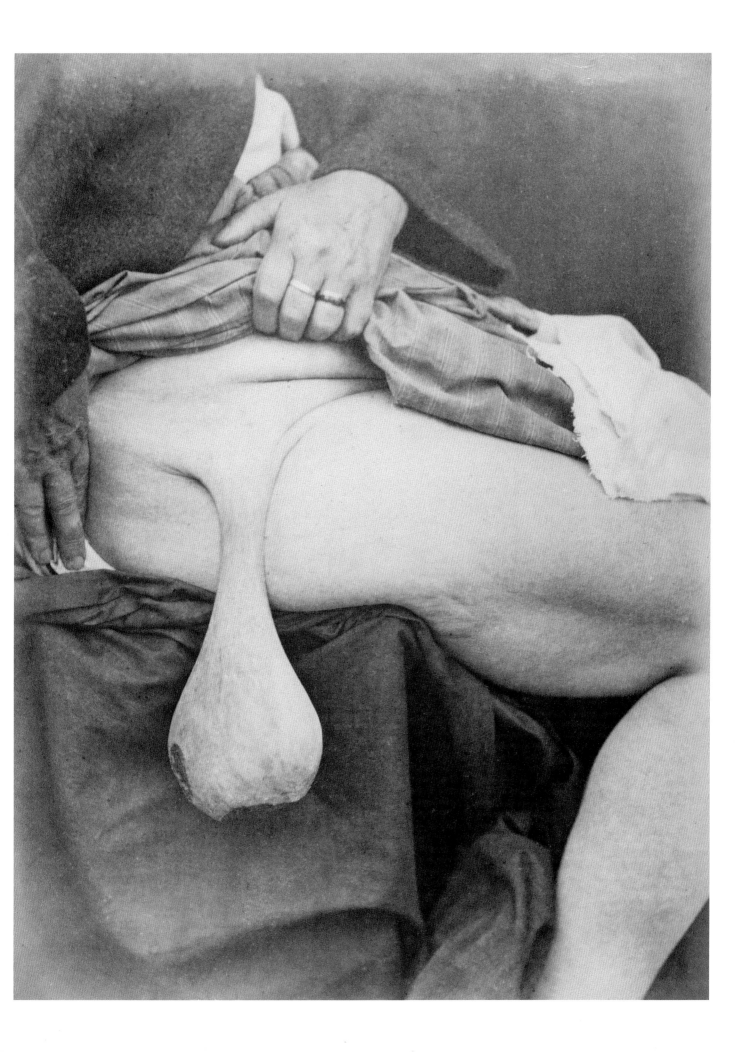

VARICELLA GANGRENOSA William F. Lockwood, MD, Baltimore, 1896

In the nineteenth century, varicella (chickenpox) was a very common childhood disease. However, dermatologists had to differentiate it from variola (smallpox), as both diseases had a wide variety of expressions. Today, the varicella virus is recognized as a member of the herpes virus family and named Varicella-Zoster Virus or 'VZV'. Varicella is basically a disease of childhood; however, it can reactivate after the initial infection. This 'reactivated VZV infection' manifests as 'herpes zoster.' While it can occur at any age, it is uncommon under the age of 50. Dermatologists today are involved in treating the secondary manifestations of herpes zoster, which can be quite serious. Varicella can now be controlled by vaccination; prior to that development it was a deadly disease, as this case indicates. Dr. Lockwood presented this photograph and history in the 1897, *Archives of Pediatrics*:

A female child, two years of age, was admitted to the Home of the Friendless, October 13, 1896... She was well and had never been sick... There were several cases of chicken-pox at the home at her time of her admission. November 13th, she was sent to the infirmary with the eruption on her face and body... The next day a wide zone of dusky redness occupied nearly the whole surface of the trunk. This dermatitis, with irregular borders, extended from about the level of the nipples to the waist... Around many of the varicella marks within this area a rapid ulceration immediately began. Both within the dermatitis area and outside of it, the contents of many of the vesicles became hemorrhagic on the second day. At the same time bleeding began from the mouth and nose, and continued during the child's illness... The skin over the right groin was puffed up with a large effusion of blood forming a huge bleb. Blood was extravasated in the skin over the pubes and genitals... The spots of gangrene varied from that of a pea to a surface measuring one inch by two inches. Their depth varied also... The deeper spots showed a dry, hard, black eschar in the center, an ulcerating border and elevated inflamed rim. Some of the largest spots of gangrene occurred outside of the dermatitis area - the largest on the inner side of the elbow... The child emitted an extremely foetid odor, which was only partly controlled by applications. Its restlessness and ill condition made a satisfactory examination of the chest impossible. Death occurred on the eighth day and was due, it seemed, to broncho-pneumonia. No Autopsy (was performed).

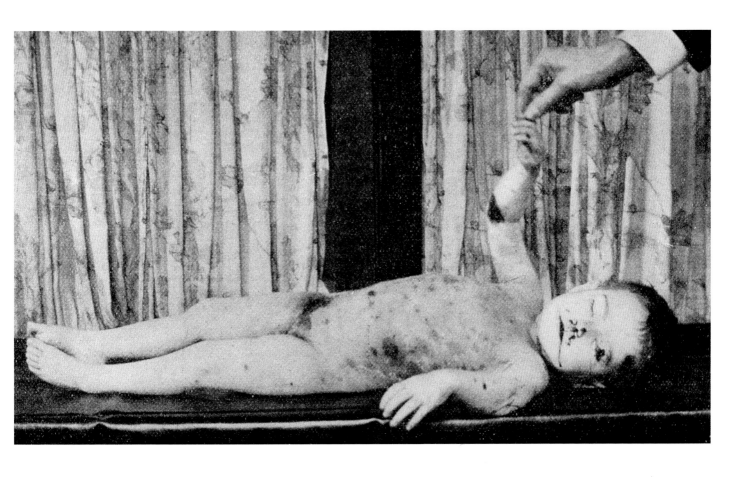

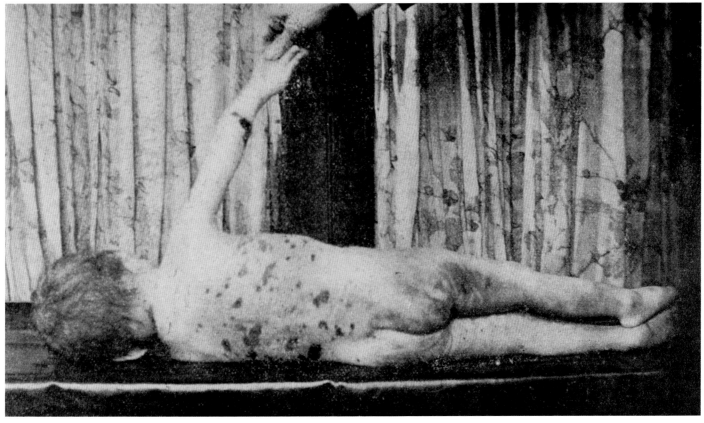

DERMATITIS VENENATA DUE TO CHRYSAROBIN George Henry Fox, MD, New York, 1900

Chrysarobin ointment was one of the most popular dermatological therapies in the last quarter of the nineteenth century. It was a miracle drug, providing one of the few valid specific therapies. Though not without complications, it was used in a variety of conditions. George Henry Fox published this image amongst the section on medication and toxic substance reactions in his *Photographic Atlas of the Diseases of the Skin*. He notes:

Dermatitis from the local use of chrysarobin in the treatment of psoriasis, chronic eczema and other skin diseases is an incidental effect which is as unavoidable as it is undesirable. When used in the form of an ointment and well rubbed into infiltrated patches it seems almost impossible to prevent the surrounding skin from becoming inflamed if the best results of this most valuable remedy are attained. A diffused redness is first noted and this often spreads to parts beyond the area to which the ointment has been applied. In certain cases an unexpected and painful congestion of the skin is occasioned with severe itching, swelling of the glands, slight fever and loss of sleep. When the application of the drug is discontinued the bright scarlet hue of the inflamed skin gradually changes to an Indian red tint. In a few days more or less desquamation occurs and soon a skin of normal whiteness is left. Upon the face chrysarobin should be used with great caution, if at all. Owing to the danger of exciting a severe conjunctivitis. Even when used elsewhere the patient should be cautioned against rubbing the eyes while any ointment remains upon the fingers. Upon the scalp the remedy is usually objectionable on account of the purplish color of the hair which is apt to result from its continued use. The plate shows all that is left of numerous discs of psoriasis after the use of a chrysarobin ointment. Instead of red or scaly spots upon a white background of normal skin, the reverse is seen. The infiltrated discs have become smooth and white and present a strong contrast with the red staining of the surrounding skin.

Chrysarobin not only stained the skin, but clothes, and almost any other item in contact with it. Strange as it may seem to us, this was an important consideration, for many clinic patients had only one or two sets of clothes.

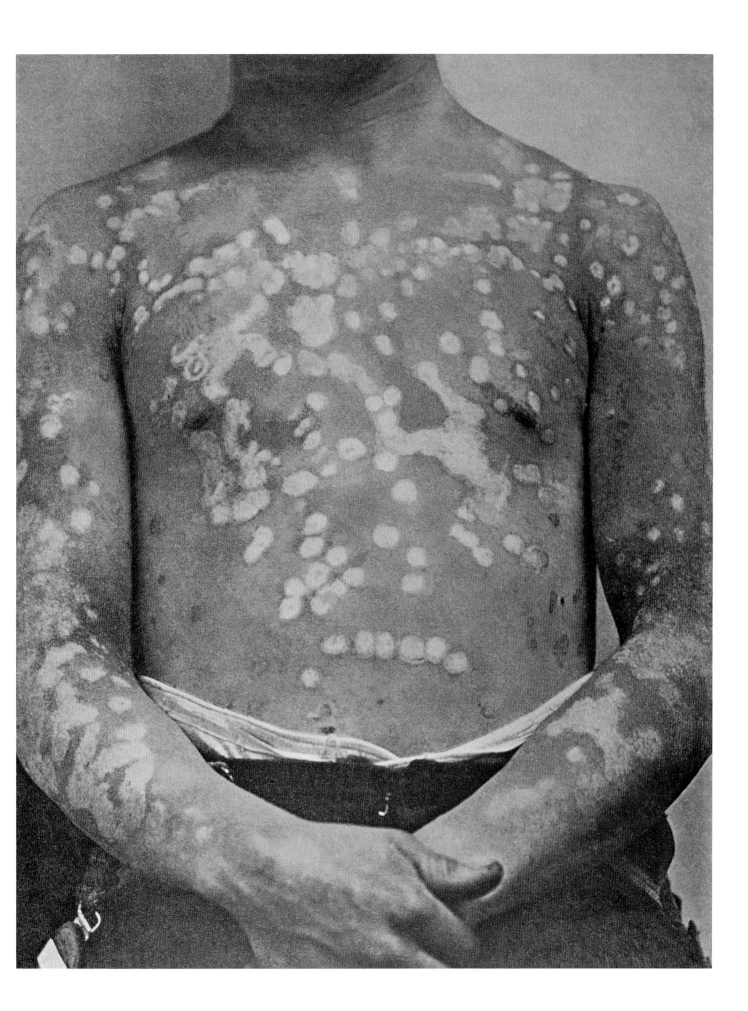

PEMPHIGUS FOLIACE Alexandre Lacassagne, MD, Lyon, circa 1897

This photograph from Lacassagne's album illustrates a typical case of an advanced stage of 'pemphigus foliacé', characterized by intense redness and desquamation of the entire skin. During the nineteenth century, pemphigus in all its forms was "a disease of uncertain cause." Now they are recognized to be autoimmune reactions. Each form has specific autoantibodies that produce the characteristic pattern of the disease. Dependent on the etiology, pemphigus foliaceus is generally divided into four subsets. Idiopathic and drug related reactions are the most common type. Even with modern therapy, the erythrodermic and exfoliative forms, as seen here, can be fatal. In 1844, Pierre-Louis-Alphée Cazenave, MD (1795-1877), published the first description of pemphigus foliaceus in *Annales des maladies de la peau et de la syphilis*, "Pemphigus chronique, générale; forme rare de pemphigus foliacé; mort; autopsie; altération du foie." It was later known as Cazenave's disease. A pupil of Laurent Biett, MD (1781-1840), he became one of the leaders of dermatology at the Hôpital Saint-Louis. Cazenave's landmark 1828 text and his editorship and authorship of the first French dermatological journal made him one of the most respected dermatologists of the first three-quarters of the nineteenth century. The 'waste basket' term 'pemphigus' was clarified by the differentiation of the forms of bullous eruptions during the late nineteenth century by Vienna's Ferdinand von Hebra, MD (1816-1880), and others. In 1888, George Henry Fox described the current state of understanding:

The term pemphigus was formally applied to every eruption of bullae from whatever cause and the affections of widely different nature, and variable prognosis were accordingly grouped under one head… Three varieties of pemphigus are commonly described. They are acute…chronic…and…foliaceus… In pemphigus foliaceus we have generally a severe case of ordinary pemphigus in which tense bullae form, but in which the epidermis becomes raised in masses by a serous discharge and dries in large whitish flakes, somewhat resembling mealy pie-crust. The disease usually progresses from bad to worse, the desquamation increasing and painful fissures form, which renders difficult all movement on the part of the bed-ridden patient. While in young persons recovery may be hoped for with proper treatment, in adults and especially in the aged, a fatal result is unfortunately the usual termination… Treatment: In the foliaceous form it is often necessary to keep the patient oiled from head to foot to lessen the cracking.

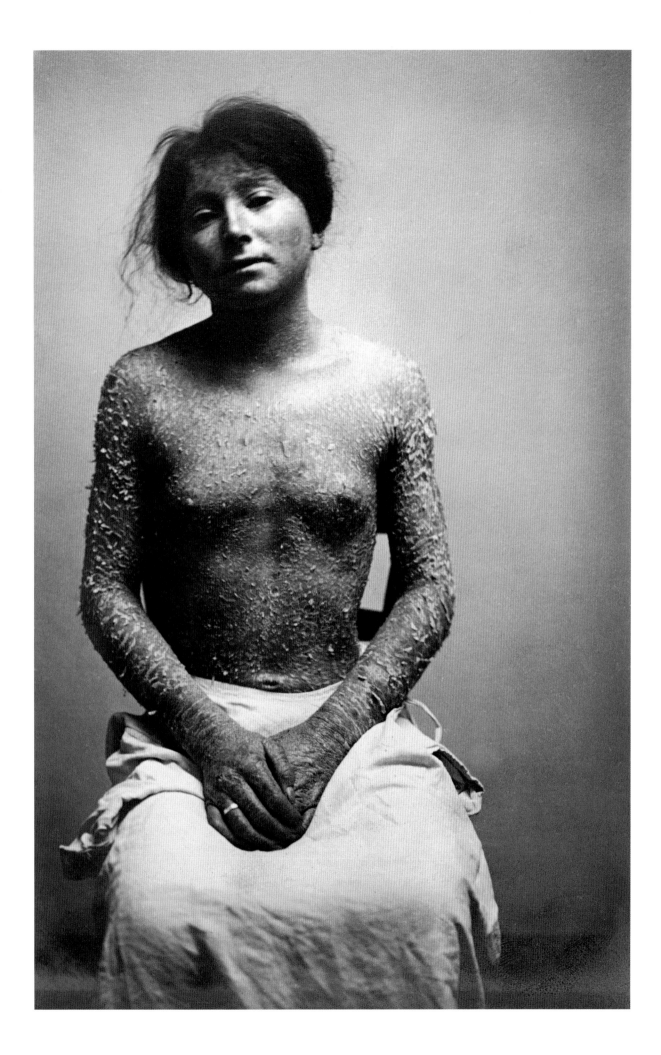

PAGET'S DISEASE OF THE NIPPLE Edmund Lesser, MD, Bern, 1894

In 1874, English surgeon Sir James Paget, MD (1814-1899), identified a new condition in *St. Bartholomew Hospital Reports*, "On disease of the mammary areola preceding cancer of the mammary." Paget recognized the eczematous condition of the nipple (and occasionally areola and surrounding skin reaction) to be associated with neoplastic disease. Classically, the involved area of the nipple is typically scaly, erythematous and occasionally ulcerated with crusting. The disease is a red flag of a mammilary carcinomatous condition and occurs in 4% to 12% of breast cancers. Dermatologists were often consulted with breast skin lesions as syphilis, tuberculosis and other infections could involve the nipple and breast ductal system. The condition now became recognized as involvement of the nipple by a ductal carcinoma. Awareness of Paget's disease allowed a correct diagnosis and treatment without untoward delay. In 1894, the same year Lesser's book was published, William Halsted, MD (1852-1922), chief surgeon of Johns Hopkins Hospital, published the development of his radical mastectomy, a procedure that would save thousands of women's lives. Paget's disease of the nipple had been found to be associated with ductal carcinoma in situ, so these patients could certainly be saved by proper surgery.

This photograph of Paget's disease of the nipple documents the extremes of disease patients often endured. Edmund Lesser, MD (1852-1918), published this image in the eighth edition (1894) of *Lehrbuch der Haut-und Geschlechtskrankheiten für Studirende und Ärtze*. The recognition of this disease placed a new burden on the 'modern' dermatologist. Lesser astutely recommended to practitioners that amputation of the breast was the necessary treatment of Paget's nipple disease. He also noted the association of extramammary Paget's eczematous skin disease, that occurred in the scrotum and penis, was similarly associated with carcinoma. Surgeon and dermatologist Henry Morris had previously identified these conditions. In 1877, Paget described a chronic inflammation of the bones - osteitis deformans. It is more common than the nipple-skin condition and also bears the name 'Paget's disease.'

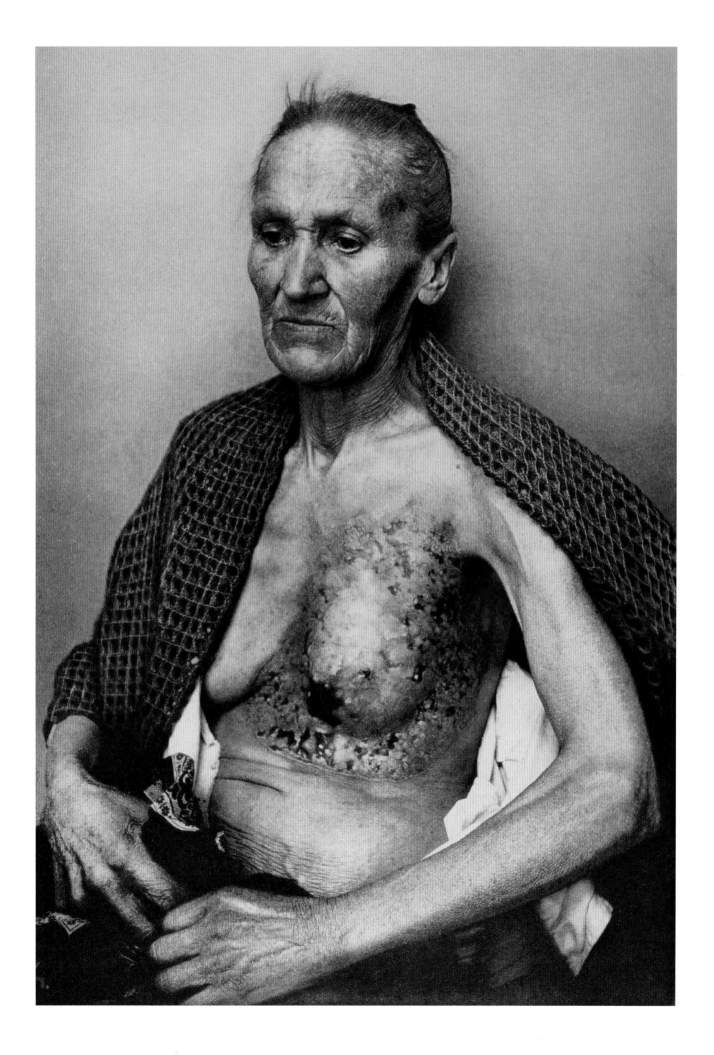

FIBROMA CUTIS George Henry Fox, MD, New York, 1900

This photograph of a patient with 'fibroma cutis' was sent to George Henry Fox, MD, for publication in his 1900 edition of *Photographic Atlas of the Diseases of the Skin* by physician W. A. Gibson of Michigan. Fox described the condition and treatment:

The man was a laborer and the tumors had been slowly multiplying for many years. Though having no effect upon his general health, their number and size interfered with ordinary manual labor. Fibroma cutis is a growth of connective tissue which gives rise to tumors of varying size and appearance. These are painless and benign in character. A very common form of the disease is the small, hemispherical nodule of firm consistence, often seen upon the face and known as naevus fibrosus. Multiple fibromata of larger size are commonly found upon the trunk. The smaller tumors are rounded and sessile, but as they increase in size they manifest a tendency to grow pedunculated, and the larger ones, on account of their weight become pendulous. While some of the smaller tumors present a certain degree of firmness the larger ones are always flaccid and pouch-like, and pressure with the finger shows that there is a thinning of the corium at the base… The cause of this fibrous growth is unknown. Many patients with multiple fibroma are small, poorly developed, and weak, and the disease may occur in successive generations. The treatment of fibroma consists solely of removal of the tumors…The small excrescencies…can best be treated by means of a sharp, curved scissors…slight hemorrhage…can be checked by touching the cut surface with a stick of silver nitrate… The firm, rounded fibroma so often occurring upon the face can be best treated by means of an electrolytic needle. This should transfix the growth…being introduced at one or more points according to the size of the tumor. This method will cause the growth to shrivel, and perhaps become necrotic… The blackish crust which forms will usually fall in a week or ten days.

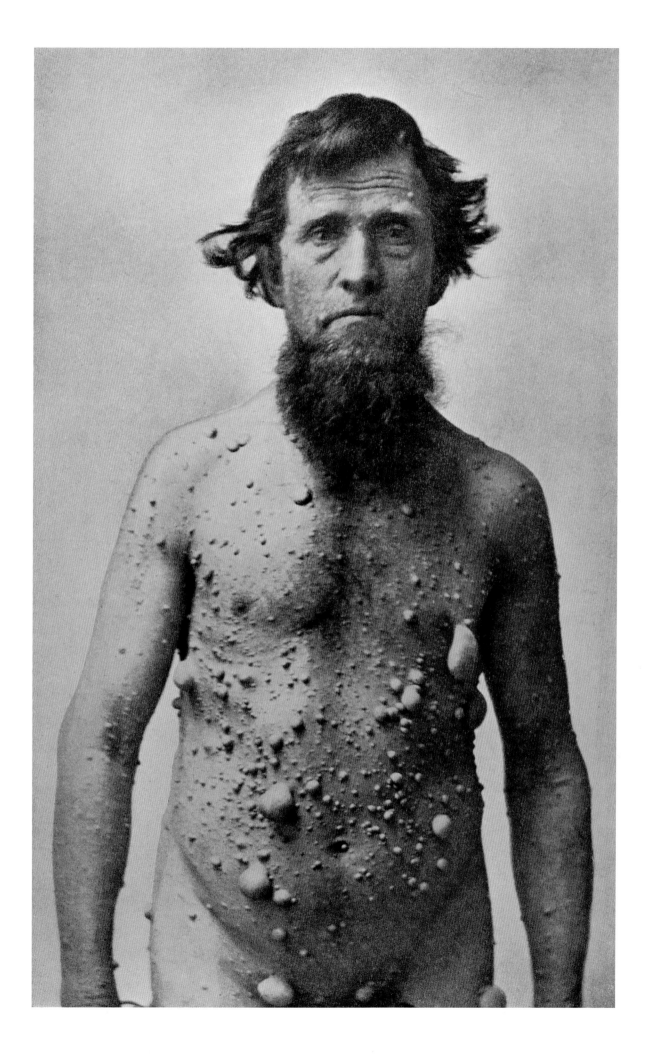

NAEVUS VASCULAIRE Alfred Hardy, MD & A. de Montméja, MD, Paris, 1868

In their 1868 atlas, *Clinique photographique de l'hôpital Saint-Louis*, Alfred Hardy and A. de Montméja attempted to present as widespread a photographic representation of the diseases encountered by dermatologists. Among the 50 photographs of syphilitic and non-syphilitic diseases presented were two images of vascular tumors. Hardy describes treating some of these tumors by doing a primary smallpox vaccination into the lesion, causing inflammation, scarring and obliteration of the lesion. He describes the vascular lesions:

> The deformities of the skin that involve the vascular system are of three varieties, which are: venous spots, vascular nevi and fungoid type nevus tumors. We have little to say about venous spots, their color varies from bright pink to a wine color. They make no projection beyond the skin, and they are not the site of any specific symptoms, but their coloration can vary and increase in intensity through temporary congestions… These stains are congenital and most often are not removable. Some however do not last and disappear a few months after birth. Others diminish in intensity little by little… The vascular nevi are composed of small regular vascular tumors alone or grouped to form a breast like protuberance and sometimes they resemble certain fruits such as strawberries or raspberries. The coloration varies from pink to brown and the nature of the vessels that come together to form these small tumors has an effect on their color. The color pink or light red belonging to arterial nevi, the color brown or purplish indicates that the tumor is formed by venous vessels. Mixed intermediate color corresponds to arterial-venous tumors formed by two types of vessels. The vascular nevi are can lead to abundant tissue or sometimes hemorrhages. These tumors are generally aggressive but they can disappear spontaneously. In these cases the projection collapses and leaves a small grey wrinkled spot. Another mode of healing consists of gangrenous changes, we see this most often in children. It begins with the appearance of a small grayish dot that spreads out over the tumor, after a few days, the scab detaches leaving a small ulcer with distinct edges. The ulcer heals slowly leaving a scar with a depression, sometimes protruding or looking like a keloid. I have witnessed several times diagnostic errors committed that resulted in ulcers being treated as if they were persistent (infectious ulcers) but were really, the result of a resolving nevi. The treatment of vascular nevi are exclusively surgical. You can destroy them with ligature, cauterization, excision, and vaccination of the tumor. I have seen positive effects of this last method applied on non-vaccinated subjects. The adhesive inflammation that develops obliterates the arteries and the other vascular tissue. The tumor is transformed into a white scar with a small depression… When the nevi are voluminous and large they are called 'tumor fongueses sanguine', and they are part of surgery and need not be addressed here.

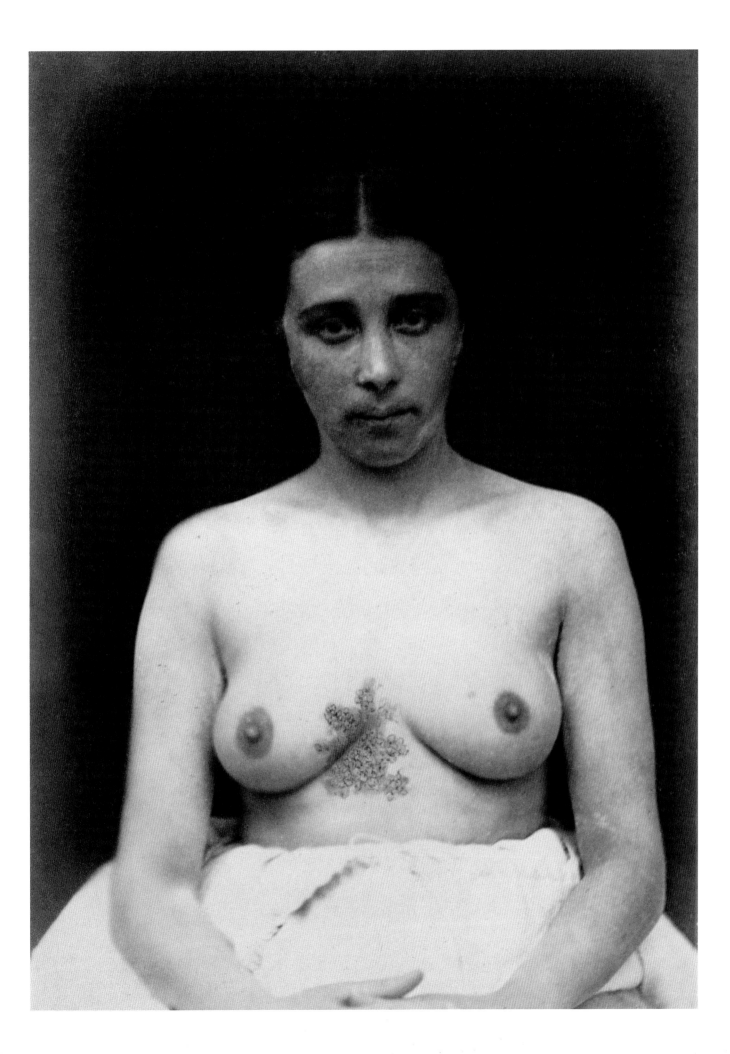

MORPHOEA Henry G. Piffard, MD & Robert M. Fuller, MD, New York, 1890

Modern dermatology was created in the nineteenth century as practitioners identified, categorized, and named diseases. During this century, several diseases were recognized to be stages, variants, or different forms of the same underlying pathological processes. Morphoea and scleroderma were acknowledged as two such associated conditions. Many early observers described an abnormal area of localized skin firmness. In 1854, Thomas Addison, MD (1763-1860), identified the localized area of skin pathology as a form of 'keloid.' However, it was England's leading dermatologist, Sir William James Erasmus Wilson, MD (1809-1884), who designated the condition as circumscribed scleroderma and suggested the name morphoea. By the end of the century, morphoea was readily identified by dermatologists and featured in texts and atlases.

This photograph was taken by Henry Piffard, MD, and presented in his 1891, *A Practical Treatise on Diseases of the Skin*, but the story was written by R. M. Fuller, MD. Piffard gave credit to Fuller on the title page, stating "Assisted By." Of the 50 full plate photographs and 33 text images, Fuller supplied only one image, but he was responsible for four of the articles, including this one on morphoea. Fuller notes:

> This patient was presented to the New York Dermatological Society by Dr. S. Sherwell. Morphoea, formally called Addison's keloid is a chronic cutaneous affection, characterized by the appearance of one or more discrete spots or patches, usually isolated and roundish in form, pinkish in color, and slightly elevated when hyperemic and hypertrophic, surrounded by a tinted or violaceous border later becoming whitish, anemic, atrophic, and slightly depressed; and in the early stage, may be seen small streaks of dilated blood vessels... In its advanced stage, morphoea is so characterized that its diagnosis is easily made. Sometimes, however it is so very like scleroderma that it is difficult to differentiate between them. In scleroderma the patches are usually symmetrically distributed, and the affected skin is hide-bound, or cannot be lifted up into a fold by the fingers, and feels hard. In morphoea the patches are asymmetrically distributed, and the affected skin feels soft or firm...the patches are often distinctly circumscribed, and confined to a limited area.

Scleroderma, the name derived from words meaning 'hard skin,' is a progressive autoimmune disease of connective tissue. It is characterized by the formation of scar tissue (fibrosis) in the skin and, in systemic cases, in various organs of the body. The fibrosis creates hardening and thickness of involved areas. Today, morphoea is still considered "localized or circumscribed scleroderma." It is, however, recognized as a disease spectrum involving a wide range of dermal sclerosing processes. While its cause is unknown, it can be associated with numerous conditions including various viral diseases, pregnancy and tick bites. Piffard's photograph depicts the classic image of the disease.

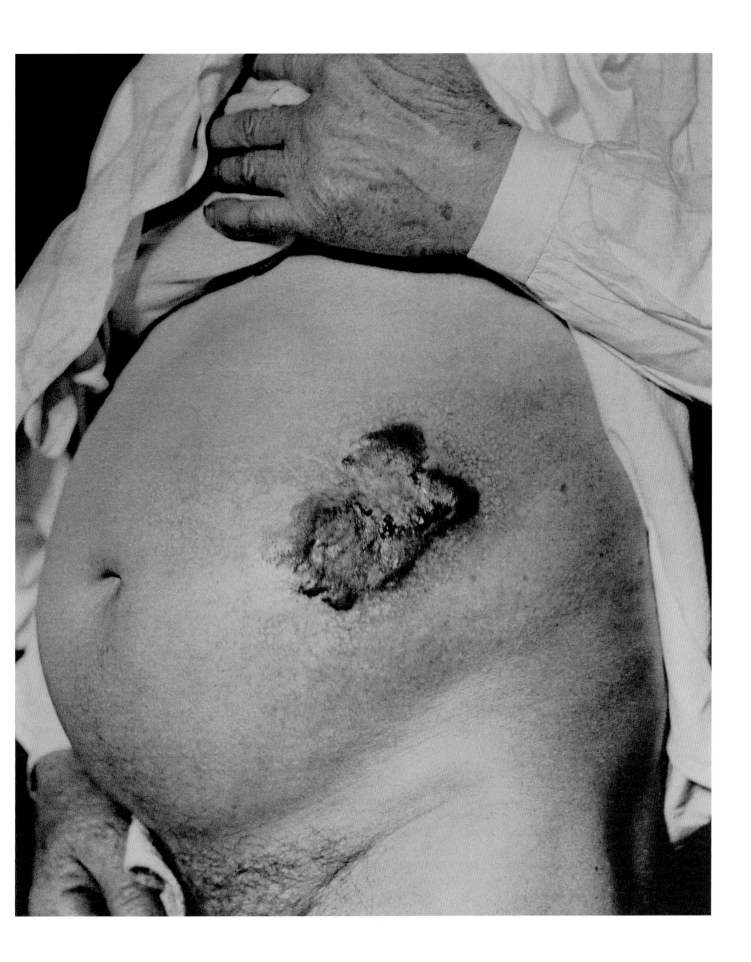

ROSEOLA MACULOSE Alexandre Lacassagne, MD, Lyon, circa 1898

This photograph from Lacassagne's album shows the mildest form of cutaneous syphilis, syphiloderma maculosa, also known as roseola syphilitica or erythema syphiliticum. The image reflects only the slightest hint of the disease. Patients with this form of syphilis sometimes ignored the mild skin reaction because, except for the 'rash', it was symptomless and eventually resolved. Dermatologist William S. Gottheil provides a good description of the level of knowledge regarding this specific syphilitic state in his 1900 text:

The erythematous or macular syphilide, is the commonest general cutaneous manifestation of the disease, and is sometimes the only one. It appears from the third to the tenth week after the advent of the chancre and being unaccompanied by itching, pain, or desquamation, is often not noticed by the patient. It shows itself as lentil- to fingernail sized, non-elevated, and usually discrete spots; but sometimes the eruption is more or less confluent, giving rise to a general mottling of the integument. Its seat is on the trunk, and it is especially noticeable upon the back; the face nearly always escapes. Its color is at first pale rose red, and fades away completely under pressure; but later it becomes a darker hue, and yellowish-brown stains are left behind when it passes away…A later macula eruption, the roseola figurate or annulata, also occurs, in which the spots are larger and often arrange in crescentic or ring shapes, Circumscribed or confluent reddened areas occur on the mucosae coincident with the roseola.

Today, the term roseola is not associated with syphilis and is reserved for a mild childhood exanthema, which had been lumped with measles, rubella and scarlet fever. In 1910, John Zahorsky, MD, described the condition "Roseola infantilis" as a distinct entity in an article in *Pediatrics* (New York). The disease is a self-limiting condition that strikes children between the ages of 6 months up to about 3 years. It starts with a prodromal high fever that lasts for 3 days and is followed by the appearance of a faint pinkish maculopapular rash. The rash fades in from a few hours to two days. Roseola is believed caused by the human herpes virus 6 (HHV-6). There are usually no complications except the high fever may result in convulsions, so that body temperature control is necessary.

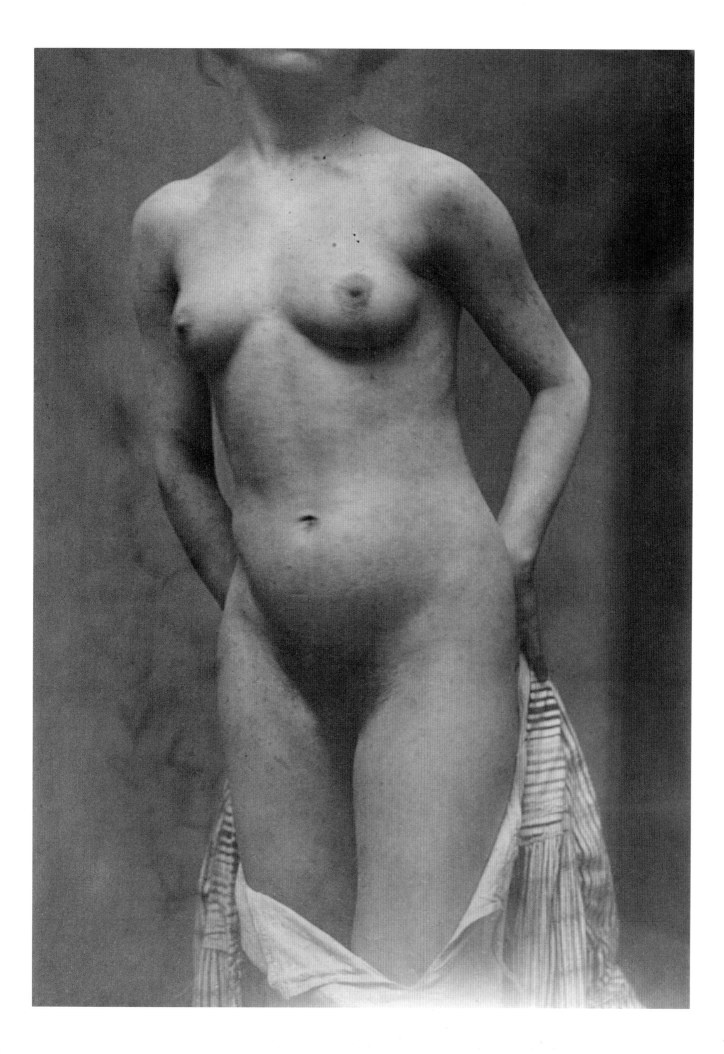

SCABIES Henry G. Piffard, MD, New York, 1891

In 1891, Henry G. Piffard, MD, published this image of scabies in *A Practical Treatise on Diseases of the Skin*. Piffard notes:

Scabies is a contagious affection of the skin characterized by the development of vesicles, pustules, and other lesions on the skin, and caused by the presence of an animal parasite, known as the *Acarus scabi*, or *Sarcoptes hominis*. The affection usually commences by the appearance of small non-umbilicated vesicles on the hands and between the fingers, accompanied with severe itching. The itching leads to scratching, and as a consequence transfer of the affection to other parts of the body with which the hands are brought into contact. Very early in the disease, then, we will find it appearing on the penis, on the breasts, and on the feet in children. From these parts it may spread over the greater part of the surface, more profusely on the anterior than posterior parts and avoiding the face and scalp. The vesicles above mentioned may be termed the primary lesions of the disease, but are usually followed in a few days by others secondary to the irritation produced by the insect, and to the effect of the finger-nails. These new lesions may be papular or pustular in character, and may even assume distinctly eczematous characters, or develop into a true eczema…

Scabies is a cutaneous disease for which the cause has been suspected for centuries. As early as the twelfth century, Avenzoar (1113-1162) identified a disease produced by little insects under the skin of the hands, legs, and feet. In 1834, Raspail, a French physician, described and demonstrated the genuine acarus and showed its connection to scabies. Fortunately, no matter how distressing the symptoms, the patient could be confidently assured of speedy relief. Piffard's treatment started with a twenty-minute warm soaking bath, then rubbed and brushed the body thoroughly with soft-soap, dried them off, then rubbed the areas with alkaline sulphur ointment with potassium iodide. The next day, new clothes were given to the patient. The entire process was repeated two or three times, as needed.

While scabies may not seem like a major dermatological entity today, for centuries, it was quite important and may have helped create a career. Ferdinand von Hebra, MD (1816-1880), professor of dermatology at the University of Vienna, became the world's leading dermatologist in the mid-nineteenth century. He made Vienna the leading dermatological educational center for decades. Hebra's fame resulted in his reclassifying skin disease, using the concept of an anatomical basis for clinical findings, building on Dr. Carl Rokitansky's (1804-1878) ideas of general pathology. When Hebra took over Vienna's University clinic in 1844, scabies was the most important dermatological entity - of 2,723 cases seen yearly, 2,197 were scabies. Hebra helped eradicate the disease.

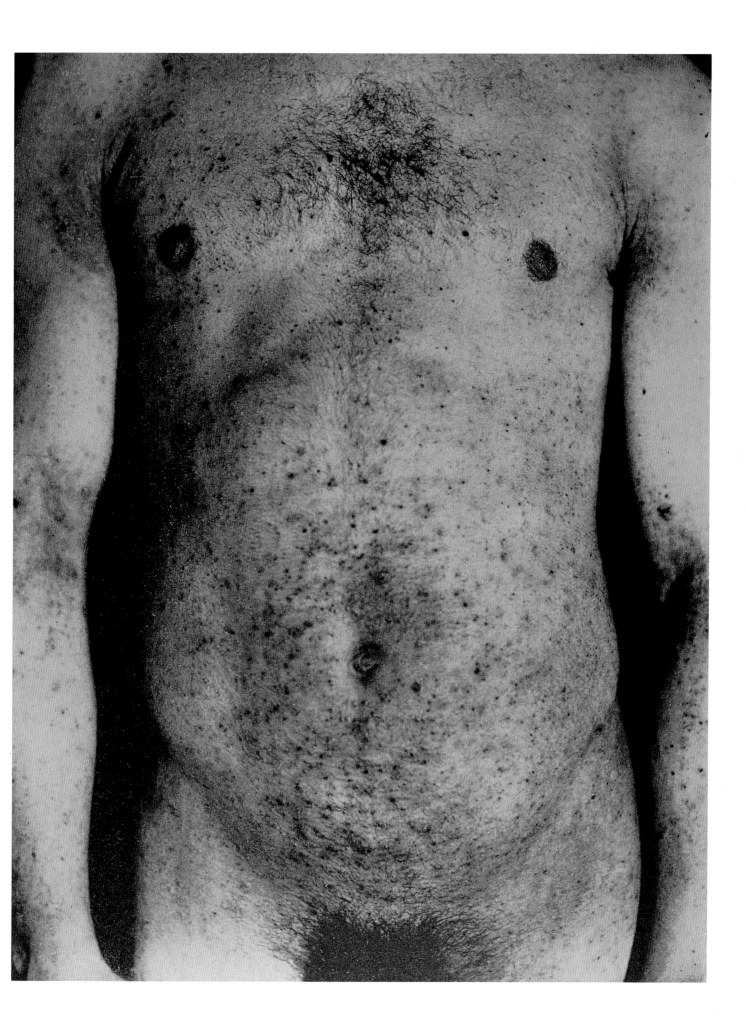

NAEVUS PIGMENTAIRE PLAN ZONIFORME Paul Spillmann, MD, Nancy, France, circa 1893

This photograph has been republished for decades in numerous dermatological and neurological texts. It illustrates the phenomenon of lesions following a particular dermatome of a spinal or cranial nerve. The term 'zona' was another name for herpes zoster. Skin lesions of various diseases that appear in a specific dermatone were called 'zoniforme.' Nevi occurred in many forms, from simple pigmented lesions to hairy or vascular forms. During the early part of the twentieth century these unilateral dermatone nevi were renamed 'naevus linearis' along with numerous other names. By mid-century the terms used were 'nevus unis lateris' or 'nevus unilateralis.' These nevi were divided into verrucous, keratotic, and the rare comedonicus type. Today, this condition is known as linear epidermal nevus. The lesions are present at birth or appear in the first few months of life.

In 1901, four physicians on the faculty of the Nancy School of Medicine, P. Haushalter, G. Etienne, L. Spillmann and Ch. Thiry, published a photographic atlas, *Cliniques médicales iconographiques*, containing images taken in Nancy in the 1880s and 1890s. There are a total of 62 large photogravure plates with 398 separate figures. The book has 25 dermatology plates each with multiple images (plates 31 to 55), for a total of over 100 dermatological photographs. The atlas is generally unrecognized as a major dermatological work. This photograph is from the clinic of Paul Spillmann, MD (1844-1914). He describes the case:

> Naevus pigmentaire plan zoniforme, in the territory of the 10th intercostals nerve. (The patient) An 18 year old girl with congenital naevi which is composed of an agglomeration of small fawn round (tawny) colored macules of varied dimensions, ranging from that of a lentil to a 50 centimes coin. They extended in the territory about the 10th intercostals nerve, roughly the size of a hand and clearly, to the median line. The lesion is a congenital malformation and the young girl has no knowledge of other such conditions in her family.

Paul Spillmann was a resident under Alfred Fournier, MD, the syphilis expert at Paris' Hôpital Saint-Louis. He returned to Nancy and became a professor of medicine. In 1880, he was appointed in charge of syphilology and headed the department until 1887, when he became professor of the medical clinic. From 1887 to 1919, 'foreign' professors held the dermatology chair at Nancy. In 1901, Paul's son, Louis Spillmann, MD (1875-1940), took over teaching dermato-venereal diseases. It was Louis Spillmann who co-authored the atlas using his father's clinical photographs. In 1919, he became the first chair in the combined dermatology and syphilology department, and then Dean of the Faculty of Medicine, in 1923. It is curious that Louis Spillmann's dermatological photographic atlas has not been noted in prior dermatological historical works. Other authors, well into the twentieth century, have used Spillmann's dramatic photographs; unfortunately, attribution was not required and authors would use any photograph that seemed appropriate.

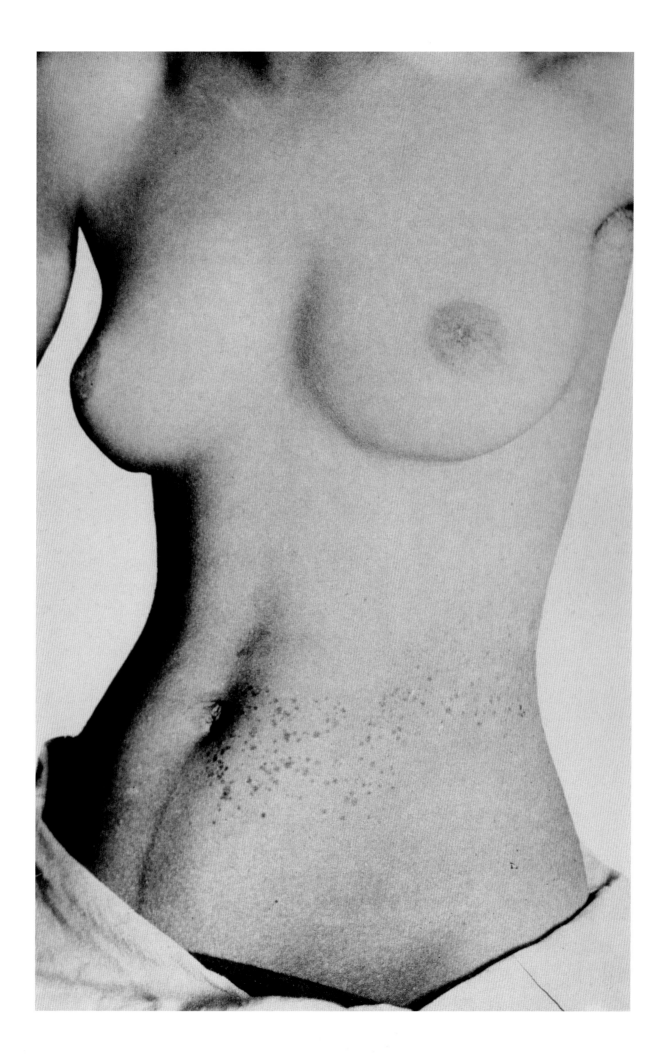

KELOID Robert W. Taylor, MD, New York, 1893

By the early 1890s, medical journals were using the half-tone photographic reproduction process to illustrate articles; however, most journals still did not include photographs within the textpage. It was the standard to present a separate page with the image, as was done with chromolithographs and photogravures. Many of the photographically illustrated articles were of exceptional conditions, such as this remarkable case of keloid reported by Robert W. Taylor, MD, in the *New York Medical Journal*, January 7, 1893. Taylor describes himself as "Surgeon to Bellevue Hospital." One month later, in the February 18 issue of the journal, Taylor notes his position as "Clinical Professor of Venereal Diseases at the College of Physicians and Surgeons, NY." In this second article, "The Pigmentary Syphilide," he presents two chromolithographs and three photographs. Born in 1842, Robert Taylor graduated from the College of Physicians and Surgeons in 1868. He specialized as a dermato-venerologist, and served as an officer of the Dermatological Society of New York. In the preamble to his case presentation he notes Maury's case of keloid (see *Back*, number 3):

Up to the present time, according to my reading, the case of keloid published by the late Dr. F.F. Maury is the most remarkable on record as regards the size of the lesion… From these facts it will be seen that the case here illustrated and described is a most extraordinary one, and well worthy of being placed on record. N.C. a rather light-complexioned colored woman is twenty-three years old, born in the United States and the mother of three children. She is perfectly healthy, came of good stock… When she was about ten years old she suffered many hardships, and was the drudge of the family, who lived in Virginia. The patient was required to go into the woods for fuel, and, having no clothes on above the waist to protect her, was frequently stung and torn in linear stripes by the briars and bushes through which she had tediously and guardedly to make her way. In the excoriations and bruises thus produced undoubtedly originated the irritative process which resulted in much marked fibro-cellular new growth, as may be seen, nearly encircling the patients waist… We will consider the tumors from above downward… (The tumor in her ear) like the rest, is of dark-brown color, mottled with very black spots and patches… This tumor is the fourth of its series… The first one began…about eight years ago… It was removed seven years ago… Tumor number two developed in two years… Four years ago it was removed, and was promptly followed by tumor number three, which in turn was removed two years ago…it was soon followed by a fourth new growth… It must weigh about…a pound… The pedunculated, lobulated, and disc-like tumors on the anterior aspect of the hypogastric region and the lateral portions of the trunk are so naturally shown, that little descriptive text is necessary…these tumors make a marked impression upon those viewing them. To some they give the impression at first that the woman's bowels have extruded, and in the minds of others the resemblance to a mass of large beef kidneys is suggested… A predecessor to these mammoth tumors was removed twelve years ago… These tumors on the back have suggested to several gentlemen the resemblance of a copperhead snake coiled up…the trunk tumors…began in a congeries of pea-size masses, fused together, and developed into the lesions depicted. During the growth of these tumors pain was not present until they had reached such a size that they had become burdensome. Then, probably from traction and upon pressure, pain of a dull aching character was felt, for which the patient sought relief in small but repeated doses of morphine… It has long been well known that the negro race is peculiarly liable to the various forms of connective-tissue new growth. I have been told by surgeons who have much to do with operations upon negroes, that in general they have a fear, even when the wound made is small, that it will be followed by keloid growth… As regards treatment, these growths as far as practicable will be removed, not with the idea of a cure, but as a palliative measure, to rid her as much as possible of her burden, and to relieve her of her pain and discomforts.

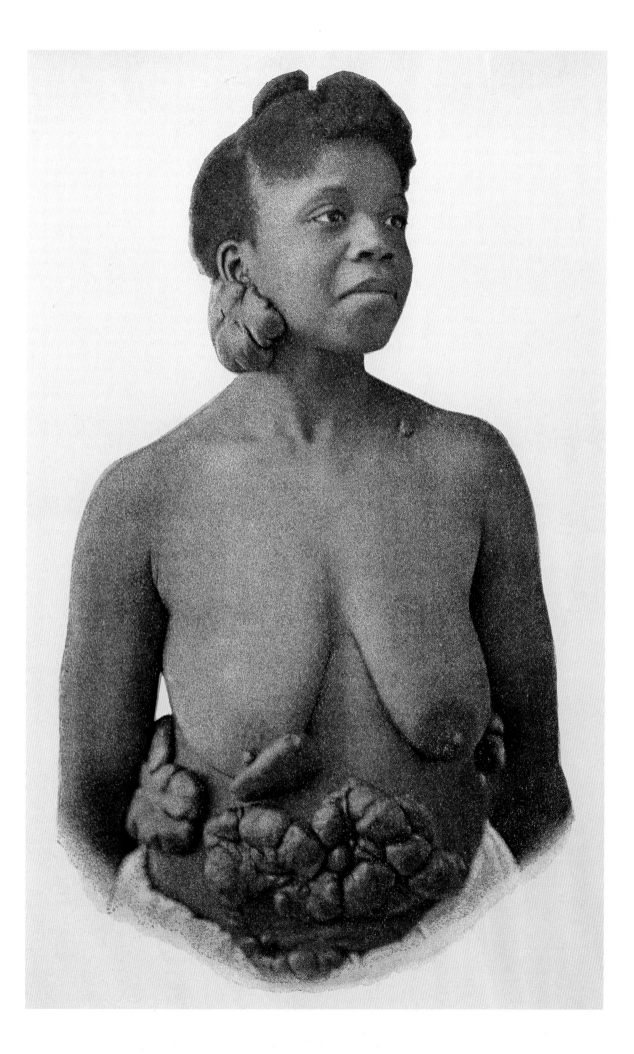

MYCOSIS FUNGOIDES Alexandre Lacassagne, MD, Lyon, circa 1896

When Lacassagne photographed this patient, he used a dramatic lighting effect to emphasize the disease, mycosis fungoides. Photographing an entire patient highlighted the conditions with which patients lived. In this era of few specific efficacious therapies, physicians often recorded every measurable aspect of a disease and patient in an attempt to find a variable leading to a breakthrough in etiology or therapy. For much of the nineteenth century, weather, especially air temperature, was recorded by physicians. The general belief was 'miasmas' and 'bad air' were the cause of disease. After the discovery of the germ theory of disease in 1882 and the elucidation of animal vectors, such as ticks and mosquitoes, in the first decade of the twentieth century, it was recognized that temperature did matter, but only as it involved the life cycle of a vector or infectious agent.

During the twentieth century, the true nature of mycosis fungoides was discovered. It was ultimately identified as one manifestation of cutaneous T-cell lymphoma (CTCL), the most common skin lymphoma. The disease symptoms appear when the skin is infiltrated by patches or lumps composed of lymphocytes. There are various stages of this disease, which encompass an entire spectrum of neoplastic proliferations, from isolated patches and plaques to Sezary syndrome. This latter condition occurs when T-cell lymphoma affects the entire skin and is called the 'red man syndrome' because the abnormal blood cells turn the skin red (erythroderma). While mycosis fungoides is the most common type of CTCL, it is still rare, with an incidence of about one new case in a million people. A condition consisting of patch lesions has been labeled 'large plaque parapsoriasis' and may be considered a pre-stage of mycosis fungoides, if not the early indication of the disease itself. Some physicians preferred not to use the mycosis fungoides label until major diagnostic changes had occurred. Lacassagne and other practitioners took photographs of patients with mycosis fungoides as part of their effort to understand and treat this perplexing condition.

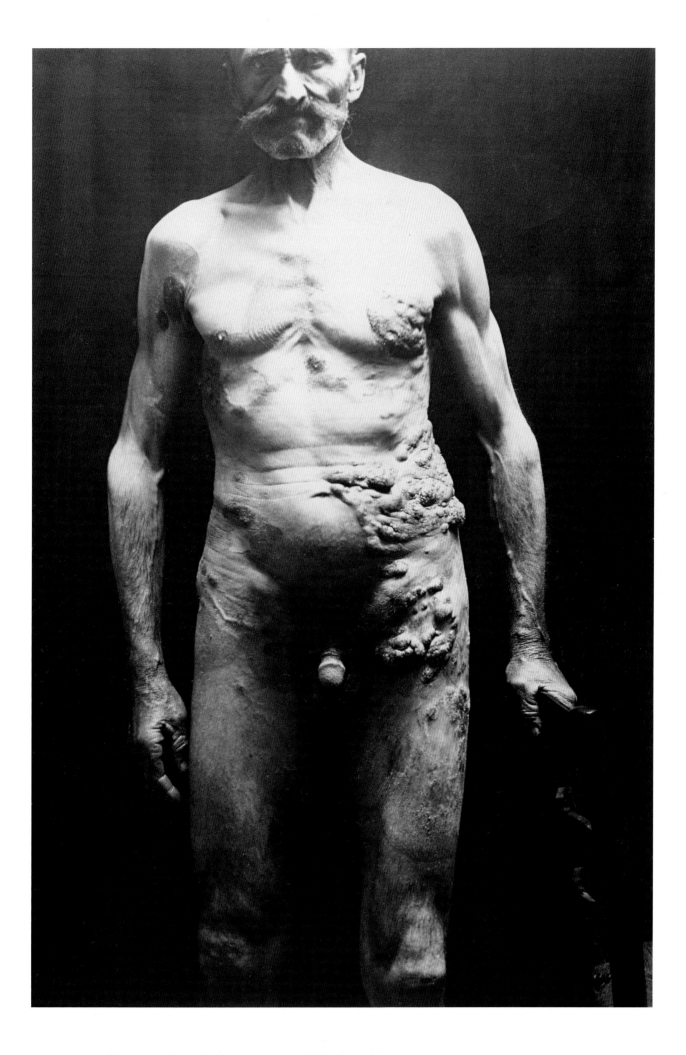

PSORIASIS ANNULATA George Henry Fox, MD, New York, 1885

This case of psoriasis annulata was presented in the 1885, *Photographic Illustrations of Skin Disease: Second Edition* by George Henry Fox. The image was one of several on psoriasis which were added to this new edition. In later editions of the atlas, such as 1888's second edition of the second series, which has 100 photographs, the reproductions of this photograph and others from prior works are less detailed. However, the photographs, which were produced for the first time for the 1885 atlas, are sharp and fresh. Fox describes the disease and the basis of treatment:

Psoriasis annulata: This case shows both scaly rings and the gyrate bands of scales which are frequently seen at the margin of a large pigmented area from which the active eruption has disappeared. In the local treatment of psoriasis, our aim should be three-fold, viz., to soothe the skin, to soften and remove the scales, and to promote the absorption of the infiltrated patches. In no disease of the skin is bathing of more importance than in psoriasis. The Turkish bath fulfills each of the three indications above mentioned, and often does more to improve the general health of the patient than the administration of drugs.

This photograph is a classic image of psoriasis annulata. The image was taken by O.G. Mason, the official medical photographer of Bellevue Hospital. Prior to his employment at Bellevue he was the chief operator at the New York photographic studio of Meade Brothers, a premier 'gallery' in the daguerreian photographic era (1840-1860). Mason's images also appeared in other noted medical atlases: in 1877, *Spinal Disease and Spinal Curvature…* by Bellevue Hospital's pioneer orthopedic surgeon Lewis Sayre (1820-1900); in 1882, *Studies in Pathological Anatomy* by pathologist Francis Delafield (1841-1915); and in 1885, *Topographical Anatomy of the Brain*, by physiologist John Call Dalton (1825-1889). The social reform movement heated up in the last decade of the nineteenth century and photography was the principal medium that attracted public attention. Dermatologist and photographer Henry G. Piffard worked with social activist Jacob Riis. O.G. Mason also assisted in the American social reform movement, taking over 1,000 photographs of New York slums, the dark side of city life and the plight of the poor. In 1892, Helen Campbell published 250 of these images as engravings in her book, *Darkness and Daylight; or, Lights and Shadows of New York Life*. Mason's principal legacies are his dramatically lit, uniquely positioned, highlighted dermatological photographs and the images he took of physicians at work at Bellevue Hospital.

In his atlases, Dr. Fox always attempted to illustrate the disease states with the most realistic and artistic examples of the malady. As he did not always have iconic images of his own patients to use, he borrowed images from other dermatologists. He used Mason as his principal photographer; however, many photographs were borrowed from Mason's own collection, which were taken for other physicians. This photograph of psoriasis annulata is beautifully lit, highlighting the lesions. Having the patient place his hands behind his head emphasizes his torso and heightens the prominence of the disease.

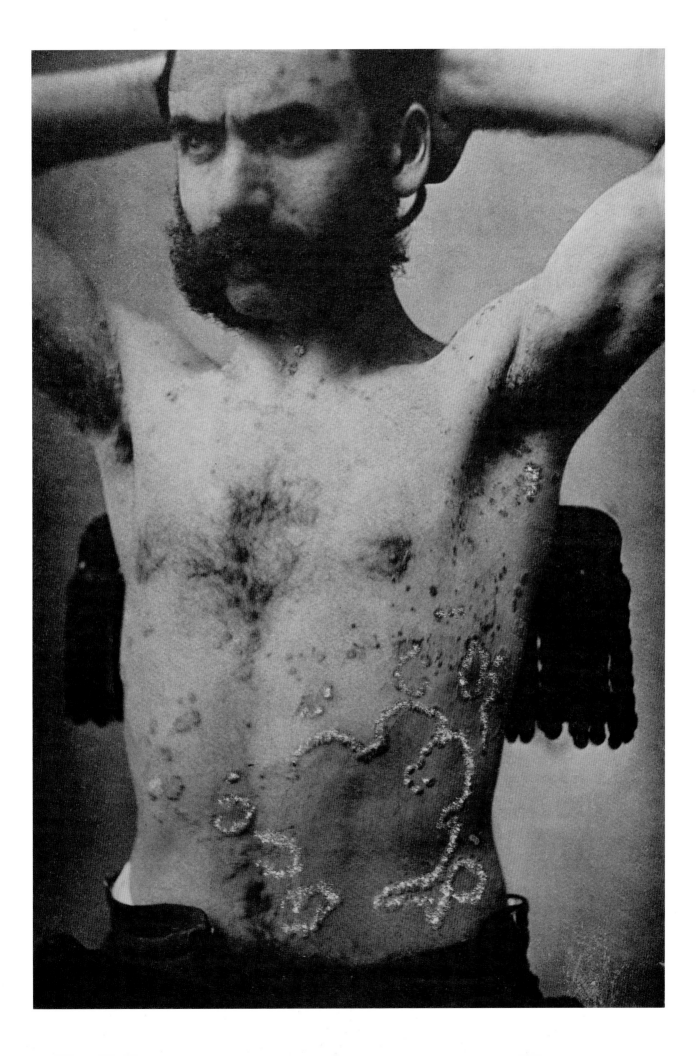

URTICARIA A. de Montméja, MD, Paris, 1873

Urticaria, more commonly known as hives, is a vascular reaction of the skin characterized by the sudden appearance of red and white swellings. They are well demarcated and transient. The swellings are localized areas of edema called wheals, which are intensely pruritic, but rarely last longer than 48 hours. This time frame distinguishes them from other skin lesions. However, in some patients, they may become chronic and recurrent for weeks, sometimes years. Almost any immunological, chemical, physical, or even psychological insult can cause urticaria, such as insect bites, pollens, inhalants, ingestants (especially drugs) and infection. Food allergies are the most common immunological cause. However, about 90% of the chronic cases of urticaria, those lasting more than six weeks, are from undetermined causes. Angioedema, a deeper swelling of the skin, occurs in 20% to 25% of all individuals some point during their lifetime. Urticaria was given its name from the reaction that occurs when the skin is touched by the plant urtica, or stinging nettle. 'Urticaria,' or nettle rash, is thought to be caused by the transmission of a venomous fluid by the minute hairs or prickles of the plant.

In the dermatology section of the 1873, *Revue médico-photographique des hôpitaux de Paris*, A. de Montméja presents and discusses cases of urticaria. He illustrates the condition with a typical patient, noting that Alfred Hardy and many others have studied and understand the condition in its various forms. Photography allowed accurate visual presentation of the various aspects of the condition. This patient, a young girl, has two different degrees of urticarial reaction. The third form of urticaria de Montméja discussed was 'edema,' which this patient did not exhibit: "The first degree consists of general cutaneous hyperesthesia and this is visible in the photograph above her breast and on her abdomen; you can see congestion produced. When you rub your nail on the skin or impress it with a coin. Very strong, very red lines are produced. The other degree and form of urticaria you see on the same subject is 'urticarial tuberose'. On different parts of the body are white spots. When you touch the spots they get bigger and more swollen."

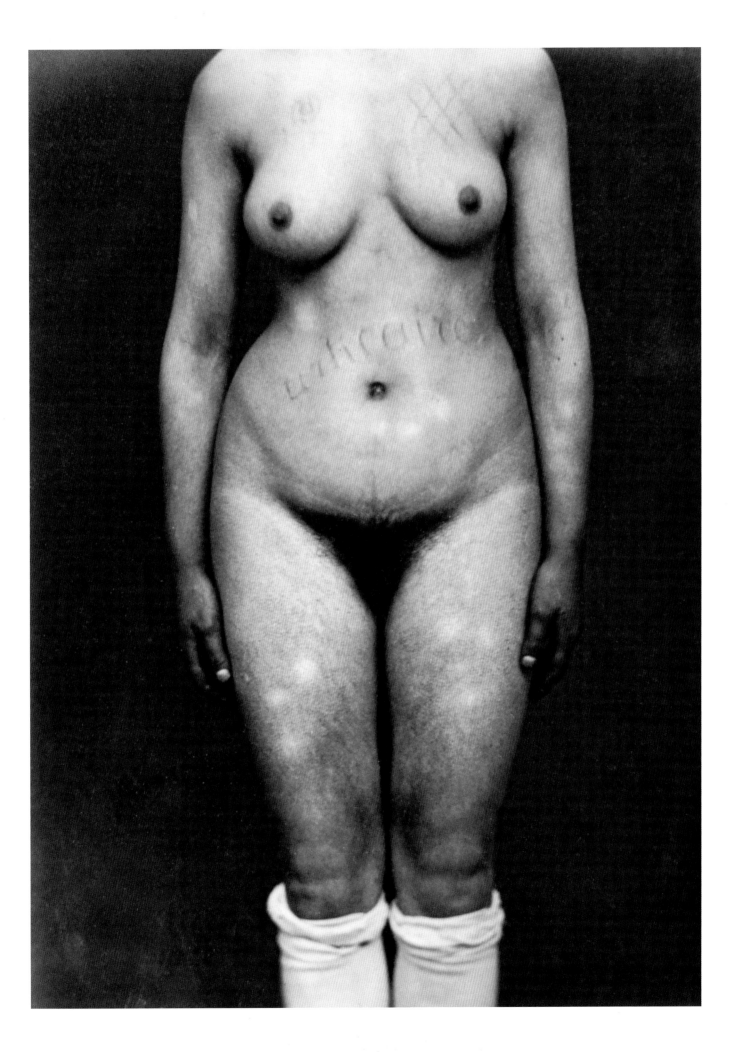

ICONOGRAPHY

Four categories of nineteenth century dermatological photography survive: 1) as images, originals and halftones in publications; 2) in donated and assembled collections in institutions; 3) as albums in private and institutional collections; and, 4) dispersed in private collections and/or held by surviving relatives and colleagues. To assist researchers, a list of the known available materials has been compiled. Not included are publications from other specialties that contained images of dermatologic conditions. This is a preliminary endeavor and hopefully will stimulate others to add to the fascinating visual history of dermatology.

NINETEENTH CENTURY DERMATOLOGICAL PUBLICATIONS WITH 'ORIGINAL' PHOTOGRAPHS

1863 Leucocythemia: An essay, to which was awarded the Bolyston medical prize of Harvard University for 1863. Howard Franklin Damon (1833-1884), *4 albumen photographs.*

1865 Photographs (Coloured from Life) of Diseases of the Skin. Alexander John Balmanno Squire (1836-1908), *25 hand-colored albumen photographs.*

1866 Casos Notables de Elefantiasis, durante su permanencia en el Brasil. José Christiano de Freitas Henriquez Junior (1830-1902), *9 albumen photographs.*

1867 Clinique photographique de l'hôpital Saint-Louis. Alfred Hardy (1811-1893) & A. de Montméja (1841-?), *A) 1867, Issued as a subscription in twelve parts with 50 hand-colored albumen photographs B) 1868, First Edition: Bound volume with 50 hand-colored albumen photographs C) 1872, Second Edition: 60 hand-colored albumen photographs D) 1882, Third Edition: 60 Woodburytypes.*

Rodent Cancer: with photographic and other illustrations of its nature and treatment. Charles Moore (1821-1870), *3 albumen photographs by Charles Heisch.*

1869 Coloured Photographs of Diseases of the Skin. Alexander John Balmanno Squire (1836-1908), *22 hand-colored albumen photographs.*

Photographs of Skin Diseases: Taken from Life. Howard Franklin Damon (1833-1884), *24 albumen photographs by A.H. Lincoln & George Moore.*

1869 Revue Photographique des hôpitaux de Paris *(1869-1872, 4 volumes)*
-75 Revue médico-photographique des hôpitaux de Paris *(1873-1875, 3 volumes)* A. de Montméja, Désiré Bourneville & J. Rengade, editors, *245 albumen photographs, about 27 related to dermatology. (Drs. Hardy, Fournier and others contributed.)*

1871 Photographic Review of Medicine & Surgery *(24 bimonthly issues).*
-72 Louis Duhring (1845-1913) & Francis Maury (1840-1879), *48 albumen photographs, several documenting unusual dermatological cases.*

1873 Extirpation of a Rodent Ulcer by the Ecraseur, Plastic Operation for the Restoration of an Entire Cheek. Charles B. Brigham (1845-1903), *2 albumen photographs in* Western Lancet, *September, (reprinted in his 1876 text,* Surgical Cases... *as heliotypes.)*

Photographic Clinique: a quarterly periodical. Alexander John Balmanno Squire, Editor, *4 hand-colored albumen photographs (one issue only).*

1876 Fibromata of the Skin and Adjacent Tissues *(Read before the Suffolk district of the Massachusetts Medical Society on February 16).* Edward Wigglesorth Jr., (1840-1896), *1 albumen photograph published in* Archives of Dermatology (April).

An Elementary Treatise on Diseases of the Skin... Henry G. Piffard (1842-1910), *5 heliotype plates of photomicrographs.*

1877 Raccolta di casi clinici delle malattie della pelle e sifilitiche curate nella clinica e dispensario. Casimiro Manassei (1824-1893), *40 albumen photographs.*

1878 Lecons cliniques sur les teignes, faites a l'hôpital Saint-Louis... Charles Laillier (1822-1893), *2 photographs by dermatologist Emile Vidal, MD (1825-1893) in a special combination process involving a mechanical print overlaid with color.*

1879 Photographic Illustrations of Skin Disease. George Henry Fox (1846-1937), *A) 1879, issued as a series of 12 articles; B) 1880, issued as a bound atlas - 48 Artotype plates by photographer O.G. Mason, hand-colored by Joseph Gaertner, MD.*

1880 Tratado clinico iconografico de dertmatologia quirurgica. Primera seccion de las lecciones de clinica quirurgica. Juan Gine y Partagas (1836-1903), *3 albumen photographs.*

1881 Photographic Illustrations of Cutaneous Syphilis. George Henry Fox, *48 Artotype plates by photographer O.G. Mason, hand-colored by Joseph Gaertner, MD (second printing 1885).*

1882 Variola: A Series of Twenty-one Heliotype Plates Illustrating the Progressive Stages of the Eruption. Samuel A. Powers, *21 heliotype plates, the majority showing the daily changes in a patient with smallpox.*

1885 Photographic Illustrations of Skin Disease: Second Series. George Henry Fox, *80 Artotype plates by photographer O.G. Mason, hand-colored by Joseph Gaertner, MD (reprinted 1886, '87, '88, '90 & '92).*

Lehrbuch der Haut-und Geschlechtskrankheiten für Studirende und Ärtze. Edmund Lesser (1852-1918), *3 collotype plates (in various forms for 14 editions/printings), 4 collotype plates in 1892 edition, other editions with different photographs.*

1891 Practical Treatise on Diseases of the Skin... Henry G. Piffard, *50 full-page heliotype plates taken by his special flash technique.*

1894 Stereoskopischer Medizinscher Atlas, Albert Neisser (1855-1916), *containing stereoscopic collotype photographs.*

1896 American Journal of Obstetrics & Diseases of Women & Children, George Henry Fox, *series of dermatologic photographic articles illustrating common skin diseases of children - each with one photograuve plate and several halftones, 77 photographs in total. (10 articles in 1896 & 2 in '97).*
"Alopecia Areata." Jan. 1896, 33:1, p.1-9.
"Ringworm & Favus." Feb. 1896, 33:2, p.187-195.
"Contageous Impetigo." March 1896, 33:3, p.354-359.
"Psoriasis." April 1896, 33:5, p.490-496.
"Ichthyosis." May 1896, 33:5, p.666-667.
"Eczema." June 1896, 33:6, p.835-843.
"Papiloma Lineare." July 1896, 34:1, p.27-30.
"Naevi, Pigmented and Hairy." Aug. 1896, 43:2, p.227-230.
"Vascular Naevus." Sept. 1896, 43:3, p.548-554.
"Lupus and other Tuberculides." Oct. 1896, 34:4, p.675-681.
"Lichen Ruber and Lichen Planus." Jan. 1897, 35:1, p.73-80.
"Various Skin Diseases of Children." Feb 1897, 35:2, p.243-254.

1897 Skin Diseases of Children. George Henry Fox, *12 photograuve plates.*

Illustrated Skin Diseases: an Atlas and Textbook. William S. Gottheil, MD, *40 photograuve plates.*

1899 Atlas der Histopathologie der Haut in Microphotographischer Darstellung. Max Joseph (1860-1933) & Paul Meissner (1868-?), *Round low-power photographs, that could also be ordered as lantern slides.*

1900 Casuistique et Diagnostic Photographique des Maladies de la Peau. Dirk van Haren Noman (1854-1896), *91 tipped-in photoglyptie photographs.*

Die Photographie in Wissenchaft und Technik. R.A. Reiss, *9 dermatalogic collotype photographs.*

INSTITUTIONAL COLLECTIONS

Allgemeine Krankenhaus, Vienna
Dittrick Medical History Center, Cleveland, OH
Musée de l'hôpital Saint-Louis, Paris
Mütter Museum, College of Physicians, Philadelphia

SELECTED BIBLIOGRAPHY

Ackerknecht, Erwin H., *Medicine at the Paris Hospital: 1794-1848*. Baltimore: Johns Hopkins Press, 1967.

Adams, George W., *The Medical History of the Union Army in The Civil War*. New York: Henry Schuman, 1952.

Arndt, Kenneth, & Philip LeBoit, et al, *Cutaneous Medicine and Surgery: An integrated Program in Dermatology*. Philadelphia: W.B. Saunders Co., 1996.

Becker, William S., & Maximillian E. Obermayer, *Modern Dermatology and Syphilology*. Philadelphia: J.B. Lippencott Co., 1944.

Beeson, B. Barker, "Alfred Hardy." *Archives of Derm and Syphil*, Jan. 1930, 21:108-111.

Bordley III, James, & A. McGehee Harvey, *Two Centuries of American Medicine: 1776-1976*. Philadelphia: W.B. Saunders Co, 1976.

Brody, Harold, et al, "A History of Chemical Peeling." *Dermatalogic Surgery*, May 2000, 26:405-409.

Burns, Stanley B., & Ira M. Rutkow, *American Surgery: An Illustrated History*. Philadelphia: Lippincott-Raven Publishers, 1998.

Burns, Stanley B., *Early Medical Photography in America: 1839-1883*. New York: The Burns Archive, 1983.

Burns, Stanley B., & Sherwin Nuland, et al, *The Face of Mercy: A Photographic History of Medicine at War*. New York: Random House, 1993.

Burns, Stanley B., & Joel-Peter Witkin, et al, *Harm's Way: Lust & Madness, Murder & Mayhem*. Santa Fe, NM: Twin Palms Publishers, 1994.

Burns, Stanley B., & Joel-Peter Witkin, *Masterpieces of Medical Photography: Selections From The Burns Archive*. Pasadena, CA: TwelveTrees Press, 1987.

Burns, Stanley B., *A Morning's Work: Medical Photographs from The Burns Archive & Collection 1843-1939*. Santa Fe, NM: Twin Palms Publishers, 1998.

Burns, Stanley B., & Jacques Gasser, *Photographie et Médecine 1840-1880.* Lausanne, Switzerland: Insitut universitaire d'histoire de la santé publique, 1991.

Burns, Stanley B., *Sleeping Beauty: Memorial Photography in America*. Altadena, California: TweleveTrees Press, 1990.

Burns, Stanley B., & Elizabeth A. Burns. *Sleeping Beauty II: Grief, Bereavement and The Family in Memorial Photography, American & European Traditions*. New York: Burns Archive Press, 2002.

Colman, William P. III, et al, "A History of Dermatalogic Surgery in the United Staes." *Dermatalogic Surgery*, Jan. 2000, 26:5-11.

Cotran, Ramzi, et al, Robbins; *Pathologic Basis of Disease, 5th Edition*. Philadelphia: W.B. Saunders Co., 1994.

Crissey, John T., & Lawrence C. Parish, *Dermatology and Syphilology of the Nineteenth Century*. New York: Praeger, 1981.

Crissey, John T., Lawrence C. Parish & Karl Holubar, *Historical Atlas of Dermatology and Dermatologists*. New York: Parthenon Publishing Group, 2002.

Cummins, S. Lyle, *Tuberculosis in History: From the 17th Century to our Times*. London: Bailliere, Tindall & Cox, 1949.

Didi-Huberman, Georges, *Invention of Hysteria: Charcot and the Photographic Iconography of the Salpêtriére*. Cambridge, MA: MIT Press, 2003.

Dieffenbach, William H., Hydrotherapy: *A Brief Therapy of the Practical Value of Water in Disease*. New York: Rebman Co, 1909.

Duffy, John, *The Healers: A History of American Medicine*. Urbana, IL: University of Illinois Press, 1976.

Editors, *Harrison's Principles of Internal Medicine, Thirteenth Edition*. New York: McGraw Hill, 1994.

Editors, *Zur Geschichte der deutschen Dermatologie*, Berlin: Grosse Verlag, 1987.

Fox, Daniel, & Christopher Lawrence, *Photographing Medicine: Images and Power in Britain and America since 1840*. Westport, CT: Greenwood Press, 1988.

Fox, George Henry, *Reminiscences*. New York: Medical Life Press, 1926.

Friedman, Reuben, *A History of Dermatology in Philadelphia*. Fort Pierce Beach, FL: Froben Press, Inc., 1955.

Frizot, Michel, *The New History of Photography*. Koln, GR: Könemann Verlagsgesellschaft mbH, 1998.

Garrison, Fielding H., *An Introduction to the History of Medicine, With Medical Chronology, Suggestions for Study and Bibliographic Data*. Philadelphia: W.B. Saunders Co., 1913.

Gilman Sander, "The Jewish Body: A 'footnote.'" *Bull Hist Med,* 1990, 64:588-602.

Harvey, A. McGee, *Science at the Bedside: Clinical Research in American Medicine, 1905-1945*. Baltimore: Johns Hopkins University Press, 1981.

Hunter, Donald, *The Diseases of Occupations*. London: English Universities Press Ltd., 1955.

Joseph, A., E. Burnett & R. Gross, *Practical Podiatry*. New York: First Institute of Podiatry, 1918.

Jussin, Estelle, *Visual Communication and the Graphic Arts: Photographic Technologies in the Nineteenth Century*. New York & London: R.R. Bowker Co., 1974.

Kelly, Howard & Walter Burrage, *Dictionary of American Medical Biography*. New York: D. Appleton & Co., 1928.

Kiple, Kenneth F., *The Cambridge World History of Human Disease*. New York: Cambridge University Press, 1993.

Lesky, Erna, *The Vienna Medical School of the 19th Century*. Baltimore: Johns Hopkins University Press, 1976.

Lévy, Gérard & Serge Bramly, *Fleurs de peau, Skin Flowers: The photographic work of a dermatologist in Lyons in the Thirties*. Munich: Kehayoff, 1999.

Lewi, Maurice J., *Textbook of Chiropopdy*. New York: School of Chiropody of NY, 1914.

Major, Ralph, *Classic Descriptions of Disease*. Springfield, IL: Charles C. Thomas, 1948.

Maulitz, Russell, & Diana Long, *Grand Rounds: One Hundred Years of Internal Medicine*. Philadelphia: University of Pennsylvania Press, 1988.

Morton, Leslie T., *A Medical Bibliography (Garrison and Morton): An Annotated Check-List of Texts Illustrating the History of Medicine*. London: Grafton Books, Andre Deutsch Ltd., 1970.

Neuse, Wilifred, et al, "The History of Photography in Dermatology: Milestones From the Roots to the 20th Century." *Archives of Dermatology*, Dec. 1996, 132:1492-1498.

Otis, George A., et al, *Medical and Surgical History of the War of the Rebellion, six volumes*. Washington, DC: Surgeon General's Office, 1870-1888.

Packard, Francis R., *History of Medicine in the United States*. New York: Hafner Press, 1973.

Porter, Roy, *The Greatest Benefit to Mankind*. New York: W.W. Norton & Co., 1997.

Pusey, William A., *History and Epidemiology of Syphilis*. Springfield IL: Charles C Thomas, 1933.

Pusey, William A., *History of Dermatology*. Springfield IL: Charles C Thomas, 1933.

Pusey, William A., & Eugene Caldwell, *Practical Application of Roentgen Rays in Therapeutics and Diagnosis*, Philadelphia: W.B. Saunders Co., 1903.

Pusey, William A., *Principles and Practice of Dermatology, 4th Edition*. New York: D. Appleton & Co., 1924.

Quetel, Claude, *The History of Syphilis*. Baltimore: Johns Hopkins University Press, 1990.

Rothstein, William G., *American Physicians in the Nineteenth Century: From Sects to Science*. Baltimore: Johns Hopkins University Press, 1972.

Schamberg, Jay F., *Diseases of the Skin and the Eruptive Fevers*. Philadelphia: W.B. Saunders Co., 1909.

Schwartz, Louis & Louis Tulipan, *Occupational Diseases of the Skin*. Philadelphia: Lea & Febiger, 1939.

Sicard, Monique, R. Pujade & D. Wallach, *À corps et à raison: Photographies Médicales, 1840-1920*. Paris: éditions Marval, 1995.

Steiner, Paul E., *Disease in the Civil War: Natural Biological Warfare in 1861-1865*. Springfield, IL: Charles C. Thomas, 1968.

Stelwagon, Henry W., *Treatise on Diseases of the Skin*. Philadelphia: W.B. Saunders Co., 1910.

Wallach, Daniel & Gérard Tilles, *Dermatology in France, Editions Privat*. Paris: Pierre Fabre Dermmo-Cosmétique, 2002.

Weyers, Wolfgang, *Death of Medicine in Nazi Germany: Dermatology and Dermatopathology Under the Swastika*. Philadelphia: Ardor Scribendi, Ltd., 1998.

Williams, Francis, *The Roentgen Rays in Medicine and Surgery*. New York: Macmillan & Co., 1903.

Winslow, Charles & Edward Amory, *The Conquest of Epidemic Disease: A Chapter in the History of Ideas*. Madison, WI: University of Wisconsin Press, 1943.

Worden, Gretchen, *Mütter Museum of the College of Physicians of Philadelphia*. New York: Blast Books, 2002.

PHOTOGRAPHIC PRINTS IN PUBLICATIONS

The iconography presented deals only with publications that contain rare, tipped-in albumen photographs and mechanical prints. Illustrations have always been desirable in publications, and they are necessary in scientific works in order to help explain or detail concepts. Photography was immediately recognized as the most inherently credible method of illustration because of its reliability, accuracy and veracity. Almost from the day photography was first presented to the world in 1839, a method for illustrating publications with photographs was sought. Since then, phototechnology has constantly evolved; to this day new types of photographs are being created. When we think of photographs, we automatically envision a photographic image formed on paper (or perhaps a digital screen).

When photography was first developed in 1826 by Frenchman Joseph Nicéphore Niépce (1765-1833), the image was on a pewter plate. Louis J.M. Daguerre (1787-1851) worked with Niépce and in the late 1830s, produced the first practical method of photography: the daguerreotype, a highly-detailed image on a silver coated copper plate. These plates could be etched with acid and reproduced as intaglio plate engravings. In 1841, an easily-duplicated paper photograph produced from a paper negative (the calotype or salt print) was perfected by William Fox Talbot (1800-1877). It was apparent that pasting the paper photographs onto pages would solve the problem of incorporating photographs in publications. Pasted-in photographs are called 'tipped-in.' The first photographically illustrated book appeared in 1844. The development of the albumen print produced by the collodion negative 'wet plate' process in the 1850s provided a more durable image. They were called albumen prints because egg whites were used in the original formula. All early photographic processes used silver salts in a light-sensitive emulsion. In the 1860s, the first medical books with photographs were published using albumen prints, including the early dermatological atlases and journals. Many were hand-painted to create more realistic images. Unfortunately, albumen prints deteriorate and fade with time, so photographic publications from this era survive in a wide range of conditions. The images vary from rich chocolate brown to sepia to pale grayish tones that are barely visible.

During the nineteenth century, numerous photographers, printers and scientists investigated and improved the process of producing photographs on paper. Printers and publishers wanted an economical reproduced image of high quality, while artists wanted the images to express their unique vision. Hundreds of photographers and scientists worked to develop a more permanent photograph, utilizing materials other then silver in the light-sensitive emulsion. One method was to replace the silver with other materials, such as platinum, carbon tissue and gum. Another method was using special presses and pigments. The mechanical photographs that resulted ultimately became the core images of the photographic atlases, texts and journals of the late nineteenth century. The principal pigment processes were the woodburytype, albertype and photogravure. Each of these methods had numerous variations, all with different names. The images were initially hand-painted to create color photographs, but mechanical color technologies had been developed and added to the basic processes by the turn of the century.

In the late 1860s, it became possible to easily print photographic books with the development of the mechanically-produced photograph, which could be mass-produced and did not fade. Two European-developed basic processes, the albertype (collotype) and the woodburytype, were introduced into publishing in the 1870s. The two types of mechanical photograph are easily distinguishable: the woodburytype was tipped-in (as was done with the albumen print), while the collotype was printed directly onto the page. Both types of photograph were produced on a heavier stock paper than the text pages, and required special printing presses. Thus, the photographs could not appear on the same page as the printed text.

The woodburytype (called the photoglyptie in France) was invented by Englishman Walter Woodbury (1834-1885) and patented in 1866. Visually, it is one of the most pleasing types of photograph ever invented. Its tonal quality is wide and its clarity is excellent, enhanced by warm tones. It has fine definition, an absence of grain or halftone screen effects, and, most importantly, it does not fade. The atlas of Amsterdam dermatologist Dirk van Haren Noman was produced in the late 1890s using a variant of the photoglyptie.

Josef Albert (1825-1886) of Munich invented the albertype in 1869. Known as the collotype today, it had numerous variations, each with a different name: heliotype, heliograph, albert-type, phototype, collographic print, ink photo, autogravure and Artotype. These photographs could be produced with a good range of tones, but are less bright and have poorer definition than albumen prints or woodburytypes. The great advantage of the albertype was that it could be printed directly on the page with easily preset margins, thus eliminating the problems of margination and the labor involved in pasting it on the page.

Edward Bierstadt of New York City bought the rights to the albertype in America and sold licenses to other photographers. In 1870, Ernest Edwards, an English photographer, modified the albertype process, naming his modification the heliotype. Many medical books were produced using this photographic printing technique, but production costs were high because up to four different inkings were necessary. In 1878, J. B. Obernetter of Munich developed the Artotype. Several men, who formed the Artotype Company of New York, bought the American rights to this process. Edward Bierstadt was the principle operator of the firm, and the prints he produced were signed 'Artotype by Bierstadt'. George Henry Fox's early photographic atlases all carry this signature.

Halftone illustrations, produced by a grid, were introduced in the 1880s. The final modern-day halftone process was developed by Max (1857-1926) and Louis (1846-1919) Levy, and patented in 1893. Halftone illustrations and their variants are easily distinguishable from other photographic printing methods because they are produced by various sized grids: examination with a magnifying glass shows that the images are made up of fine dots of varying color. These images were considered 'photographic illustrations', not fine photographs. The advantage of the halftone was that it could be easily reproduced on the same page as print, using the same presses. By 1901, the halftone was the photographic process of choice for medical publications, and the age of 'mechanical' and 'tipped-in' photographs was over.

The photogravure was the result of the application of photography to the artist's aquatint printing method, and is among the most beautiful of all phototechnologies. The rich, colored inks that were available to all intaglio printing processes were responsible for its beauty and visual effect. Photogravures from the 1876 to 1900 era are exceptionally detailed, and can be enlarged so that details not visible to the naked eye are revealed. In the nineteenth century, such art photographers as England's Peter Henry Emerson (1856-1936) and Scotsman Thomas Annan (1829-1887) used this process. At the turn of the century, some of America's noted photographers used the photogravure process in their photographs and publications, the most famous being Alfred Steiglitz (1864-1946) in his *Camera Work*, and Edward S. Curtis (1868-1952) in *The North American Indian*. Paul Strand, Albert Langdon Coburn and other major photographers produced works as photogravures because of their inherently aesthetic properties. The photogravure and other permanent prints are considered fine 'original' photographs. Many are inherently more beautiful than the original surviving silver prints of the same image. By the 1890s, several expensive modifications had been made to the process, allowing photogravures to be printed in color. The dermatological works of William S. Gottheil are examples of the most advanced of these processes. This series presents beautiful photogravures produced by dermatologists Edmund Lesser of Germany, Louis Spillmann of Nancy, France, and New York's William Gottheil, Henry Piffard and George Henry Fox. These photogravures, along with other mechanical and silver prints used in early dermatological atlases, are today recognized as an important legacy to art and photography, as well as to the history of dermatologic education.

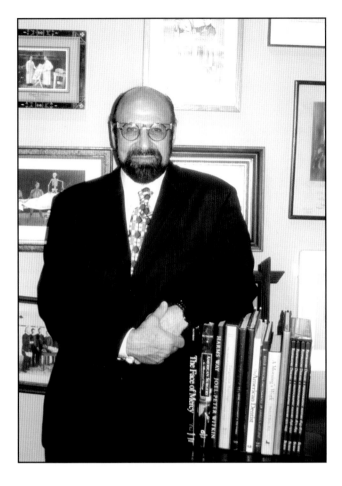

STANLEY B. BURNS, MD, FACS

Stanley B. Burns, MD, FACS, a practicing New York City ophthalmic surgeon, is also an internationally distinguished photo-historian, author, curator and collector. His collection, started in 1975, is considered the most comprehensive private historic photography collection in the world. This archive of over 700,000 vintage prints contains the finest and most comprehensive compilation of early medical photographs, consisting of 70,000 images taken between 1840 and 1940. They have been showcased in countless publications, films and museum exhibitions. The Burns Archive, his stock photography and publishing entity, is a valuable photographic resource for both researchers and the media. He is also a consultant for Hollywood feature filmmakers, as well as independent producers. Some of his film credits include, Adrian Lyne's *Jacob's Ladder*, Robert Altman's *Dorothy Parker and her Vicious Circle*, Tom Cruise's *The Others* and Al Pacino's *Looking For Richard*. France's Channel Plus created a documentary on his work as part of their *Great Collectors of the World Series*. Dr. Burns has been an avid medical historian since 1970. From 1979-81, he was President of the Medical Archivists of New York State. He has been a member of the medical history departments of The Albert Einstein College of Medicine and The State University of New York, Medical College at Stony Brook; curator of photographic archives at both The Israeli Institute on The History of Medicine (1978-1993) and The Museum of The Foundation of The American Academy of Ophthalmology. Currently, he is a contributing editor for seven specialty medical journals. Using his unique collection Dr. Burns has written ten award-winning photo-history books, hundreds of articles and curated dozens of exhibitions. His film company, Black Mirror Films, produced *Death in America*, an award-winning documentary on the history of American death practices. He is continuing his medical specialty photographic series with volumes on cardiology, psychiatry, urology, infectious disease, neurology, women's health and ophthalmology. He is currently working on several medical books and exhibitions, as well as books on criminology, Judaica, Germans in WW II and African Americans. He can be reached through his web site www.burnsarchive.com.

ACKNOWLEDGEMENTS

I am most appreciative of the members of my family who are integral parts of The Burns Archive. They have assisted me, tirelessly, in preparing this historic compilation. I especially thank my daughter Elizabeth, the creative director at the archive and was responsible for the production and design. I am most grateful to Saul G. Hornik, MS, RPh., medical advertising consultant. It was his enthusiasm and recognition of the educational importance of my medical, photographic collection, together with his tireless work that made this series of publications possible.

I want to express my sincere appreciation to several unique individuals who helped with various aspects of this project: Jennifer Frances Dinsmore, RN, Morgan Stanley Children's Hospital of New York. New York Presbyterian Medical Center, assisted with research; Lisa Barocas Anderson translated the French medical journal case histories; Mark Rowley continued my original photographic bibliography (1981) in his monograph, *Photo Illustrated Medical Literature* (2004). This work stimulated me to create a bibliographic iconography of dermatological photography. Several curators supplied information and assisted in research, offering their valuable time to help me document various aspects of dermatological history, thanks to: James Edmonson, Curator of the Dittrick Medical History Center, Case Western Reserve University School of Medicine, Cleveland; Michael Rhode, Chief Curator, National Museum of Health and Medicine, Washington, DC; Miriam Mandelbaum, Curator of Rare Books and Manuscripts, Historical Collections, New York Academy of Medicine. Several dermatologists, who are among the leading historians in the field, provided valuable contacts, sources and information. I am sincerely grateful to: Lawrence Charles Parrish, MD, founder (1973) and current president of the History of Dermatology Society, Philadelphia; Daniel Wallach, MD, founding President of the French Society for the History of Dermatology, graciously sent me a copy of his masterwork *Dermatology in France*, and introduced me to current European dermatologic historians, among them Karl Holubar, MD, professor in dermatology and director of the History of Medicine Institute in Vienna and Jacques Chevallier, MD, of Lyon, France, dermatologist and historian on the executive committee of the French Dermatological Historical Society. Much thanks to Parisian photography collector and historian, Gerard Levy, for two decades of mutual admiration and help on projects. He is a kindred soul, and his book *Fleurs de peau, Skin Flowers: The photographic work of a dermatologist in Lyon in the Thirties*, helped me sort the dermatological images of Lyon and the work of the Lacassagne family. I also want to acknowledge Daniel Glassman (President and CEO), Gene Goldberg (Senior Vice President) and the personnel of Doak Dermatologics/Bradley Pharmaceuticals, for their support and interest in this photographic history series, as well as their understanding of the educational value in using the visual history of the past as a foundation for the future.

OTHER PUBLICATIONS

Oncology: Tumors & Treatment, A Photographic History 1845-1945 (4 Volumes)

Respiratory Disease: A Photographic History 1845-1945 (4 Volumes)

Sleeping Beauty II: Grief, Bereavement and the Family in Memorial
Photography, American & European Traditions
with Elizabeth A. Burns

A Mornings Work: Medical Photographs from The Burns Archive
& Collection, 1843-1939

Forgotten Marriage: The Painted Tintype & The Decorative Frame
1860-1910, A Lost Chapter in American Portraiture

American Surgery: An Illustrated History
co-author: Ira M. Rutkow, MD

Harm's Way: Lust & Madness, Murder & Mayhem
co-authors: Joel-Peter Witkin, et al

The Face of Mercy: A Photographic History of Medicine at War
co-authors: Matthew Naythons, MD & Sherwin Nuland, MD

Photographie et Médecine 1840-1880
co-author: Jacques Gasser, MD

Sleeping Beauty: Memorial Photography in America

The American Dentist: A Pictorial History
co-authors: Richard Glenner, DDS & Audrey Davis, PhD

Masterpieces of Medical Photography: Selections From The Burns Archive
co-author: Joel-Peter Witkin

The Bristol® Gallery of Medical History (7 Volumes)

Early Medical Photography in America: 1839-1883

WWW.BURNSARCHIVE.COM